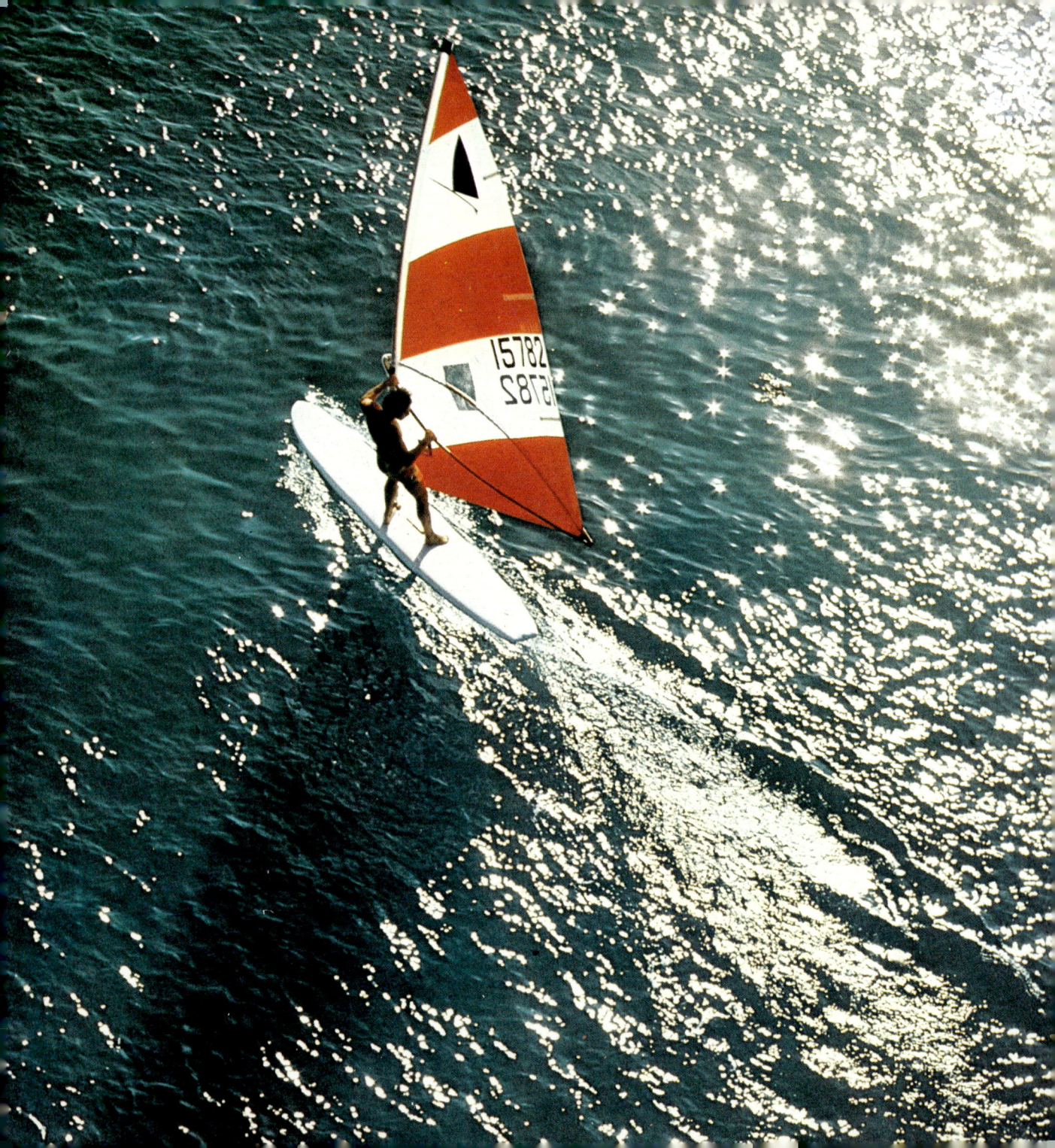

Windsurfing

Uwe Preuss, Jochen Taaks and
Karsten Kemmer

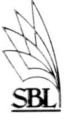 **Springfield Books Limited**

Acknowledgements

The authors and publishers would like to thank the following companies for their kind support: Mistral, BicMarine, and Gaastra.

Special thanks are also due to our friends and colleagues Sepp Winbeck, who wrote the chapters on the weather and tides, and Sigi Hofmann and Volker Möhle, who offered useful suggestions and information.

Preuss, Uwe
  Windsurfing.
  1. Windsurfing
  I. Title   II. Taaks, Jochen
  III. Kemmer, Karsten
  IV. Der Segelsurfschein in
  Theorie und Praxis. *English*
  797.1'24   GV811.63.W56
  ISBN 0–947655–05–0

Photographs on pages 94–95:
  Gunter Steinbach (10),
  German Weather Service,
  Hohenpeissenberg (1)
All other photographs: Michael Garff
Drawings: Lutz Köbele, Sabine
  Gillner and Sepp Winbeck
Layout and design: Yves
  Buchheim
Cover design: Douglas Martin
  Associates
Cover photograph: Alastair Black
Translation: Hansheinrich Barthel,
  Michael Fuchs, Anthony Rich,
  Andrew Shackleton

Colour reproduction: Arti Litho,
  Munich
Typesetting: Paul Hicks Limited,
  Oakfield Press, Plymouth,
  Devon PL5 3NA
Printed and bound in Spain for
  Paul Hicks Limited
ISBN 0 947655 05 0

Contents

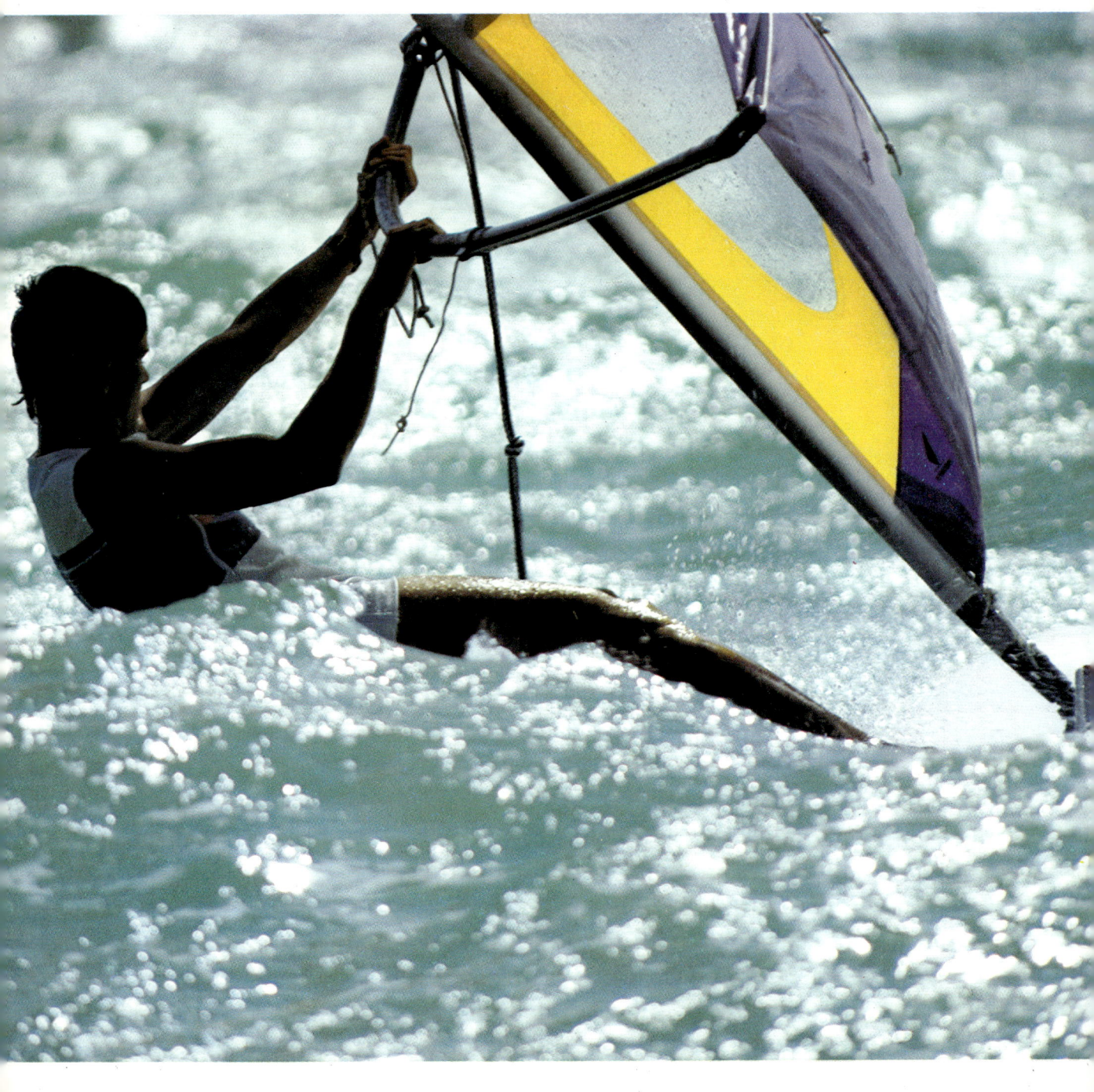

Introduction

There is a fascinating outdoor sport which ten years after its introduction has won a mass following: windsurfing.

The trend was recognisable as long ago as the late 70s, but only today can it be fully appreciated. More than half a million people — men, women and children of almost every age — practise this sport more or less regularly and with a great deal of enthusiasm. Different forms have appeared, which are similar to the two older sports from which the new sport of windsurfing developed fifteen years ago.

On the one hand, there are people sailing around on lakes close to towns, or taking part in races, on boards that resemble small boats. Both of these possibilities are also offered by sailing, one of the two roots of windsurfing. On the other hand, there is also the exciting experience of coastal surfing on tiny boards over breakers, which comes close to surf-riding, the other origin of our sport. The newcomer to this sport, just as much as the old hand, can experience both the thrill of gliding over the water and all the other sporting opportunities offered by windsurfing.

One thing that all surfers must have in common, though, is the knowledge that they are not just using a piece of sports equipment for their own pleasure; they are operating a sailing vessel. Everything you need to know in order to be able to use this vessel in a responsible manner and without endangering others can be found in this book.

In this context, it is not only important to know about regulations, laws and codes of behaviour, but above all to work constantly on improving your surfing technique, in order to be able to control the board in difficult situations, whether you have caused them yourself or whether they have occurred unexpectedly.

The best theory is useless if inadequate skill and technique prevents you from putting it into practice.

Theoretical knowledge is not useless if it helps you to avoid emergencies and dangerous situations, and to get out of difficulties should something go wrong despite all precautions.

For this reason, both the theoretical and the practical sections of this book contain more information than you need if you simply want to obtain a windsurfing certificate. In particular, the skills

Windsurfing: you can't get any closer to nature.

7

described in the practical section go beyond what you need to be able to do in order to pass a windsurfing test; it contains a series of exercises which we recommend you to try out.

Controlling the board better and being able to play with it and its potential mean quite simply that you will be able to have more fun more safely. More and more people are taking up windsurfing, although the water surfaces available are not getting any bigger. At the same time, more and more surfers want to try out more difficult conditions, and the boards are becoming faster.

There is going to be less room to move on our waterways; the interests of nature conservation have to be taken into consideration. This makes it all the more necessary for every surfer to keep his knowledge and skill up to date all the time, and to undergo tests of his knowledge and ability.

The quickest way to become proficient in boardsailing is to be taught at one of the many hundreds of sailing schools which have been set up to cope with the amazing and accelerating increase in the number of people who wish to take up the sport. There are schools all over the world at which you can learn and when on holiday you can go and learn in one of those which have perhaps warmer water than is ever available in the United Kingdom. Most of the courses run by different organisations are essentially based on the format first evolved by a man called Dagobert Benz who operated on Lake Constance and early realised that he would need to produce a "step-by-step" system in order to teach properly.

It is always the way with a new sport that the man who starts the teaching organisation must first teach a whole lot of instructors who, in their turn, can start teaching either other instructors or pupils.

Nearly all the national authorities in each country have handled matters in the same way. In the United Kingdom the Royal Yachting Association was already running many forms of training in the use of boats — dinghy sailing, cruising, powerboat handling and so on. So it was a natural step for that organisation to take up the original work and to organise some more schools, many of which have already become part of the Recognised Teaching Establishments scheme of the RYA. Whilst it is not difficult to find a teacher you are *best* advised to be taught at one of these "recognised" schools, rather than try to teach yourself by constantly falling off your board in the cold waters round our coasts.

One of the best reasons for going to one of these schools is that they all have that marvellous invention (first evolved through the IWS scheme) of a "simulator". It is virtually, in most cases, a sailboard mounted on a revolving platform which reacts exactly as a real sailboard would when on the water. So you learn at your own speed and on dry land exactly how to manage the start and the theory of sailing. Most important, you soon get the feel of where the wind is coming from and begin to understand that the wind is your vital source of power supply! It is the motive

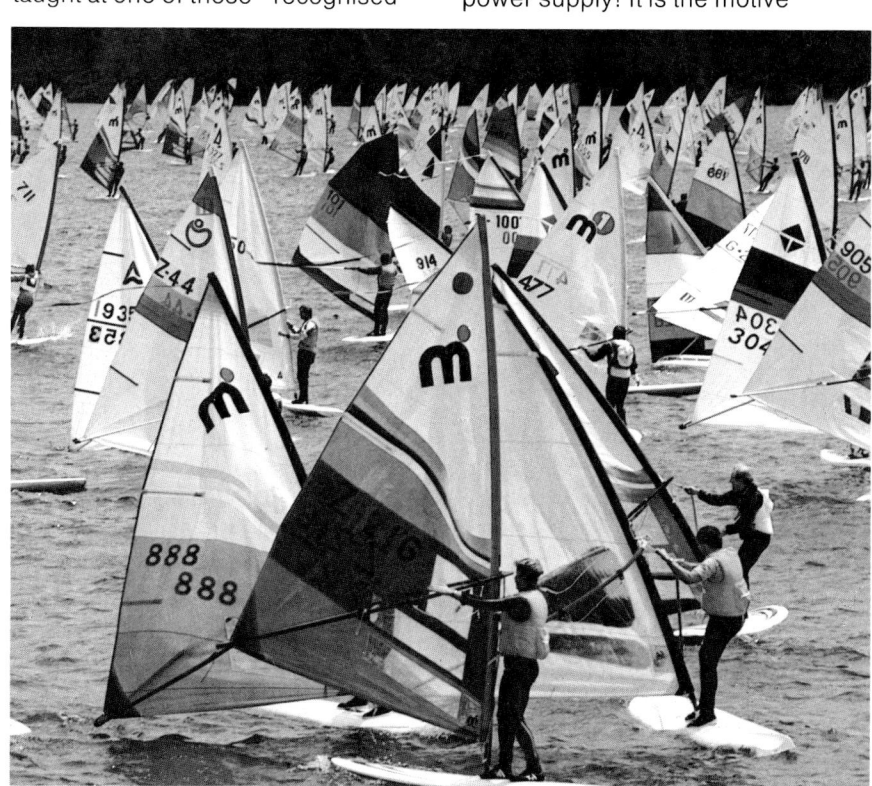

power, and you learn how to use it rather than letting it blow you where you don't want to go!

Since many of the places in the world where you can hire a sailboard require to see your certificate before they will let you on the water with their precious property it is important to obtain a certificate at an early point in your boardsailing career. Then you can make use of the many package holidays which are available to young and old to go to the warm water and warm weather and to enjoy, at the same time, a "continental" holiday.

Curriculum for the RYA National Boardsailing Certificate

The items listed below sum up the curriculum which needs to be mastered by a really competent boardsailor.
● seamanlike handling of ropes
● importance of appropriate clothing for the sport
● familiarity with the safety rules
● importance of a safety line
● behaviour under different wind and weather conditions
● how to take precautions against emergencies and in distress
● familiarity with the International Distress Signals
● how to behave during rescue
● familiarity with the Golden Rules of behaviour for water sports
● familiarity with the regulations governing transporting equipment on a car roof
● care of the surfboard

The actual RYA National

Boardsailing Scheme Awards are divided into three blocks. There is first the *Starter Course* which is part of the *National Boardsailing Award*. There is then an optional *Improvers Course*. The third block is divided into the *Advanced Open Sea Award* or, if you prefer, the *Advanced Inland Award*. The latter is quite sufficient for those who sail on gravel ponds or on such waters as large reservoirs.

The *National Boardsailing Award*, which includes the starter course, consists of the following items:
● *Swimming* (25 metres)
● *Rigging* Assembling and stowing all parts of the board and knowing their names
● *Knots* Just a few simple knots — the bowline, the figure-of-eight, and other suitable knots
● *Carrying the equipment*
● *Personal equipment and safety clothing* The effect of hypothermia and all about wetsuits and drysuits. Buoyancy aids, distress signals, flares, visibility, safety leashes, etc.
● *Simulator* Demonstrate control of board
● *Wind and weather*
● *Tides*
● *Launching and recovery*
● *Sailing* A simple triangular course including tacking and gybing
● *Self rescue*

Then there is the *Improvers Course* which includes:
● *Rigging* A more advanced syllabus including the different types of sail, selection of correct sail for conditions, the use of battens, tensioning the sails etc.
● *Harness* Introduction to the harness, harness lines and methods of attachment
● *Launching and recovery* With

board and rig assembled, doing beach and jetty starts
● *Sailing* Really improving your technique, including weight distribution, etc. and the use of various positions of daggerboard
● *Boards and equipment* Outlining the different types of board and their practical uses.

When you reach the *Advanced National Boardsailing Award* it must be taken in at least fifteen knots of wind. During the free sailing time the Instructor will pay particular attention to the style and confidence with which you execute your manoeuvres and the balance and trim of the board on all legs of the triangular courses which you will be sailing.
● *Launching and recovery* will be executed from all shores including the different lee shores
● *Sailing* will be much more advanced and you will be doing flare gybes, emergency stops and even sailing without a daggerboard
● *Rescue techniques* will be practised. As you will read in this book, towing is part of the safety programme
● *Wind and tide* will be studied in as great a depth as is discussed in this book, because it is so important for your own safety
● *Theory* will also be investigated and you will find that much which you have read in this book will be useful
● *And finally* there will inevitably be long lectures on buoyage, other water users, different types of board, their uses and limitations, etc.

Altogether, these courses will not take you very long and they will teach you a great deal.

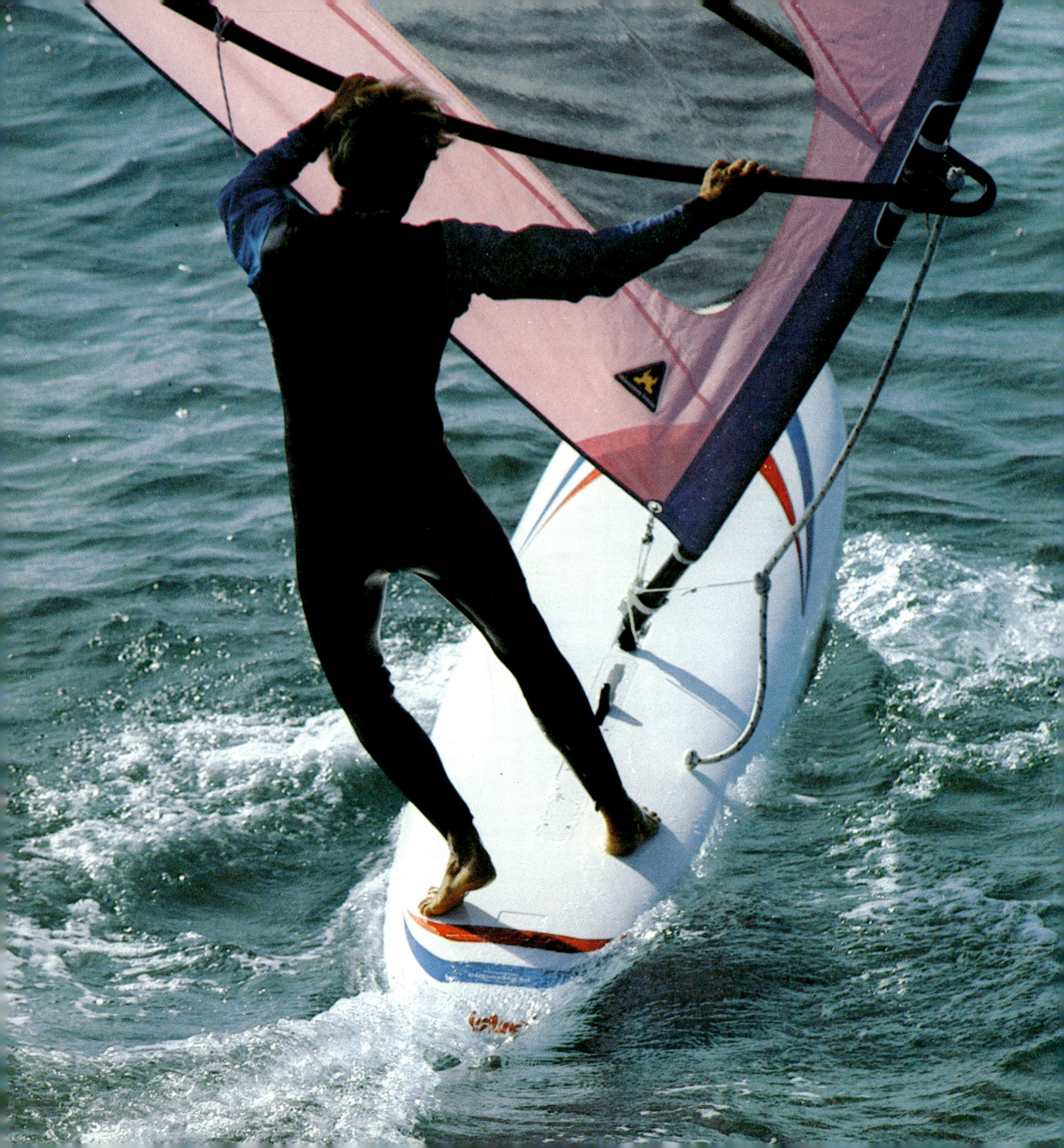

Windsurfing in practice

It is impossible, and probably undesirable, in this practical section to present in detail all the possibilities offered by windsurfing. On the other hand, we felt it was important to describe more skills than those needed by the beginner. However, we are not going to try and describe in detail the whole range of possible skills, or to explain all the different views on how to carry out particular series of movements.

On the contrary, experience has shown that in the manoeuvres described, there are clearly definable key positions, and it is enough to understand and master these. It is often sufficient to know a particular trick, and this will increase one's skill and pleasure.

For this reason, we considered it a prime necessity to present clearly and in great detail these particularly important elements in an otherwise complex series of movements. We have applied the same principle in our descriptions of other complicated matters.

This concentration on essentials is of course especially useful for those who have already learnt the basic principles of surfing and who have gained their first practical experience on a surfboard.

All the same, we have also included a clear and easy-to-follow summary of the basic skills, so that the newcomer will find answers to his questions, and will have no difficulty in preparing for this sport, which offers so many exciting opportunities.

Yachtsmen use certain technical terms, which also apply to our sport. These terms can often express an idea far more precisely than any carefully-thought-out description. Whenever these words are not explained in the context itself, they can be found in the glossary at the end of the book.

It will become apparent not only in the descriptions of the skills, the tips and exercises, but also in the illustrations accompanying them, that it is impossible to draw a clear line between beginners and advanced learners. The photographs will more or less speak for themselves. They were taken especially for this book. Unless there is a specific note to the contrary, all the demonstrations were made on allround boards, because the difference between the beginner and the advanced learner does not lie in the special equipment or in a completely different surfing technique. Everything the beginner learns can, with a little practice and experience, be transferred directly to the advanced stage.

Tacking quickly by steering with rig and edges

Assembling the rig

If you stand on the shore and examine the structure of other windsurfers' rigs, you will notice that these rigs have been set up in a wide variety of ways. Every make has its own peculiarities. With a new board, you should study carefully the accompanying instructions for its assembly. In order to get the greatest possible pleasure from your surfing and prevent damage to the equipment, you should assemble the rig in a seamanlike way. Even if you have already had some experience in assembling rigs, compare the following instructions with your own practice to make sure you have not acquired any bad habits.

Insert mast in mast sleeve

To do this, have the top of the sail (the head) lying to leeward, and insert the mast carefully in order to avoid damaging the mast sleeve.

Insert mast foot in mast, and secure with downhaul line

Insert the mast foot in the mast. Make sure that no sand gets in

between the mast and the mast foot (Illustration 1). Tie a short bowline in the downhaul line, and reeve it twice through the bowline and the tack

cringle. Finally, secure the downhaul line with two half hitches (see page 78) over the reeving (illustrations 2–4).

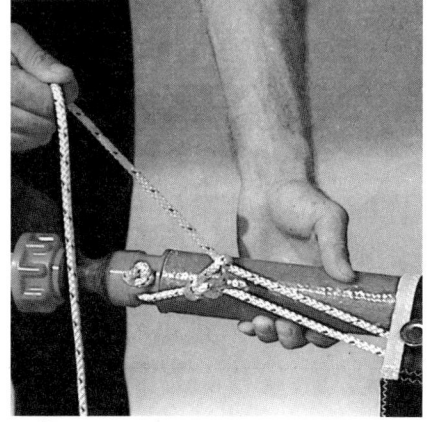

▲ 2

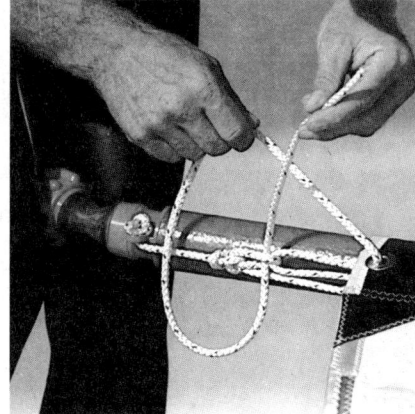

▲ 3

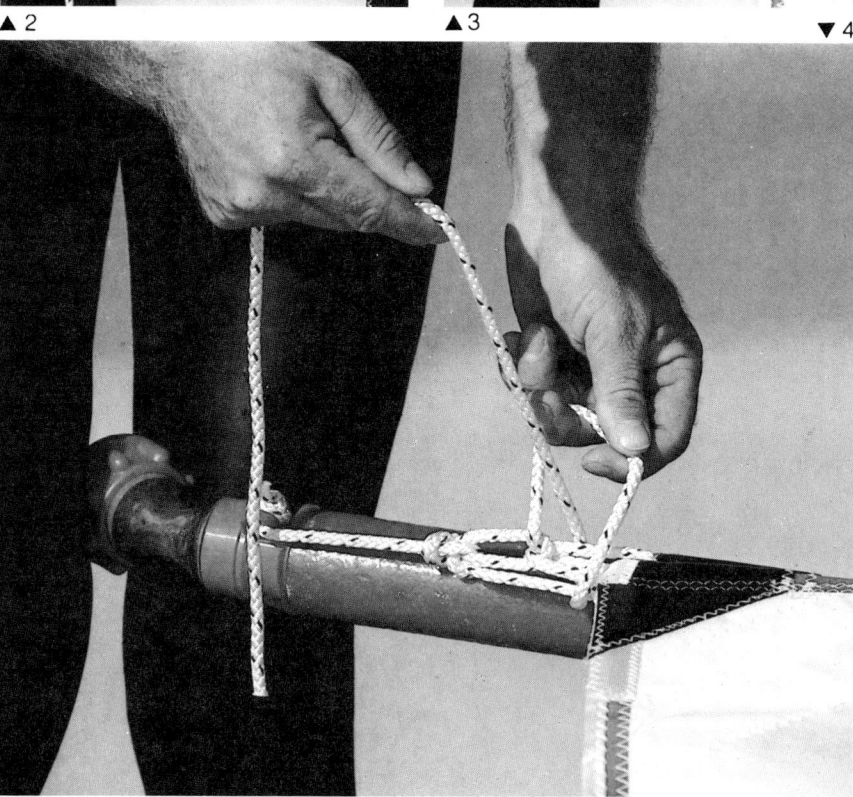

▼ 4

1

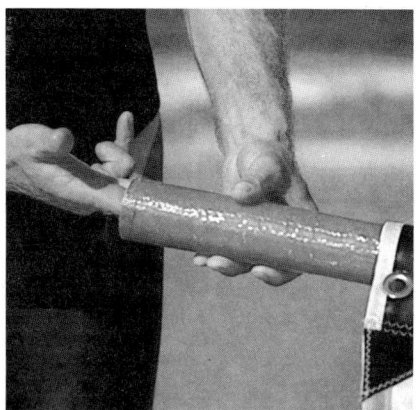

Tie inhaul line to mast at eye level

Tie the inhaul line to the mast with a rolling hitch (see page 76). Then stand the mast upright and push the hitch to eye level. Be sure to leave at least two inches' room between the knot and the top of the gap in the sail. Later, when you trim the luff (see below), you will need this room, as the mast sleeve is pulled downwards slightly in the process.

Tie wishbone to mast

Draw the inhaul line through one of the holes in the head of the wishbone, back on the same side, round the mast, through the other hole in the head of the wishbone, and finally fix it in the cleat (illustrations 1–2).

Secure inhaul line

Secure the inhaul line with at least two half hitches (see page 78) immediately behind the cleat (illustration 3).

Insert battens in pockets

The slightly notched side of the batten is held in the sail by elastic strops. Slide the batten as far in as possible, and then let the other end of the batten slide back into a pocket attached to the leech for this purpose.

Trim and secure luff with downhaul line

Trim the luff with the downhaul line, which needs to be reeved at least twice, until there are no folds left in the mast sleeve. Finally, secure it again with two half hitches over the reeving.

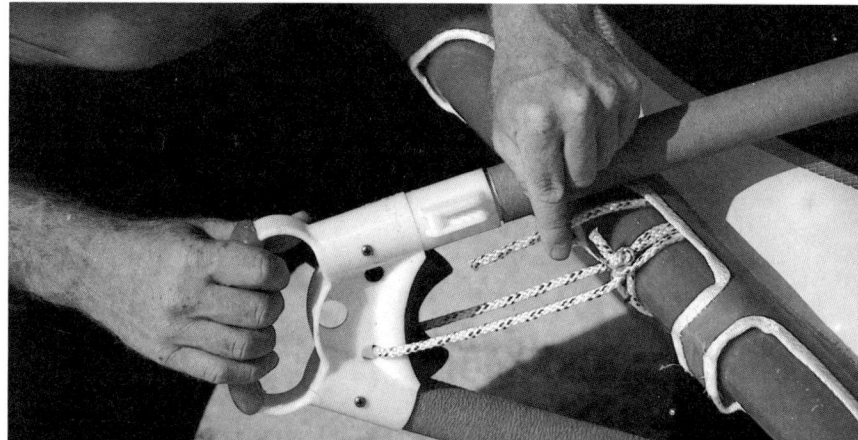
1

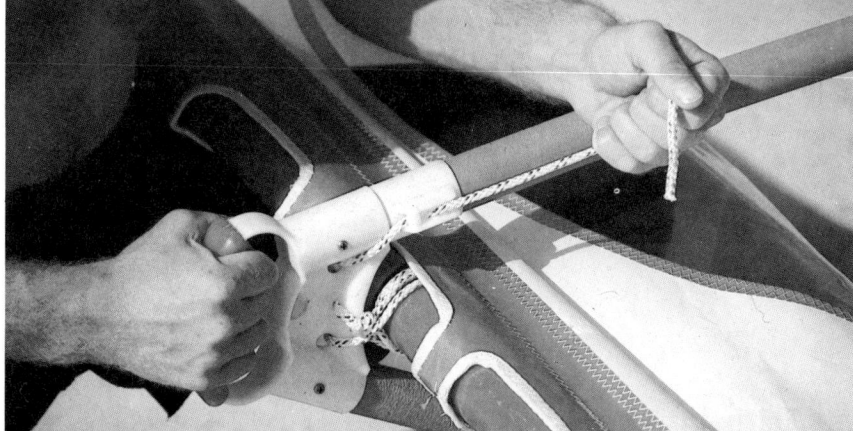
2

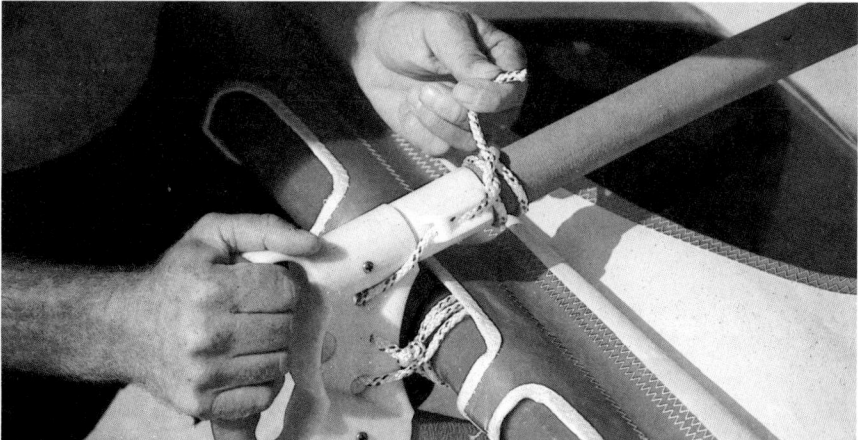
3

Attach and secure sail with outhaul line

Most instruction manuals tell you to reeve the outhaul line between the two cleats in the rear part of the wishbone and the boom end fitting (illustrations 1 and 2). However, we recommend that you attach the outhaul line to the boom end fitting with a bowline (see page 76). In this way, you cannot lose the end of the rope, and you will need less rope.

The following procedure can be recommended as an energy-saving way of attaching the sail: lay the mast at right angles to the wind, with the clew to leeward. Take hold of the sail near the clew with one hand and press the boom end against your stomach. Then pull hard, and with your free hand pull the loose part through the reeving. Take hold of the outhaul line *and* the wishbone with the same hand, and press the two together tightly. With your other hand, draw the loose outhaul line through the cleat. Secure it immediately in front of the cleat with two half hitches.

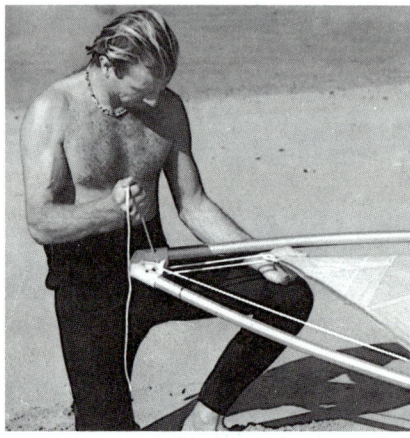

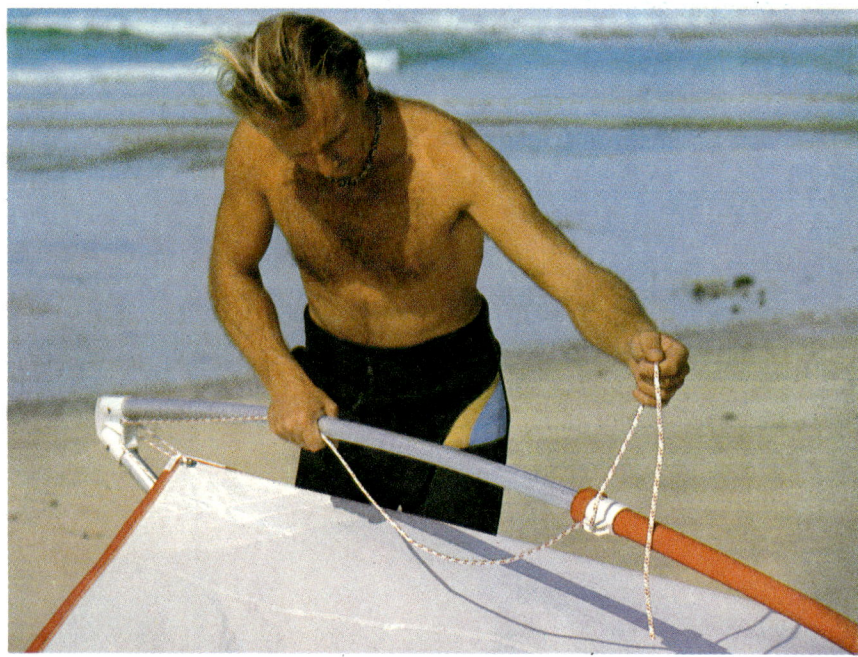

Checking the equipment

Finally, check the following points carefully.

Rig

● Are the rope ends worn (damaged)?
Yes: replace them
● Can the mast foot be turned easily?
No: dismantle and clean it
● Is there a gap between the head of the wishbone and the mast?
Yes: loosen the outhaul line, and tighten the inhaul line
● Can you see any cracks in the boom end fittings?
Yes: replace them
● Is the stopper hitch away from the edges of the gaps in the mast sleeve?
No: loosen the outhaul line and the downhaul line, loosen the rolling hitch, and slide it up or down the mast as appropriate

Board

● Is the surface slippery?
Yes: remove sun-tan oil and/or apply wax
● Is the outer skin damaged?
Yes: repair small holes or cracks (see page 79); have more serious damage repaired by an expert
● Are the daggerboard and mast foot easy to move and fix?
No: clean the base of the mast, adjust the daggerboard fitting
● Is the skeg fitted securely?
No: tighten or replace the screws

Upkeep and simple repairs to the board and the rig are described on pages 79 and 80.

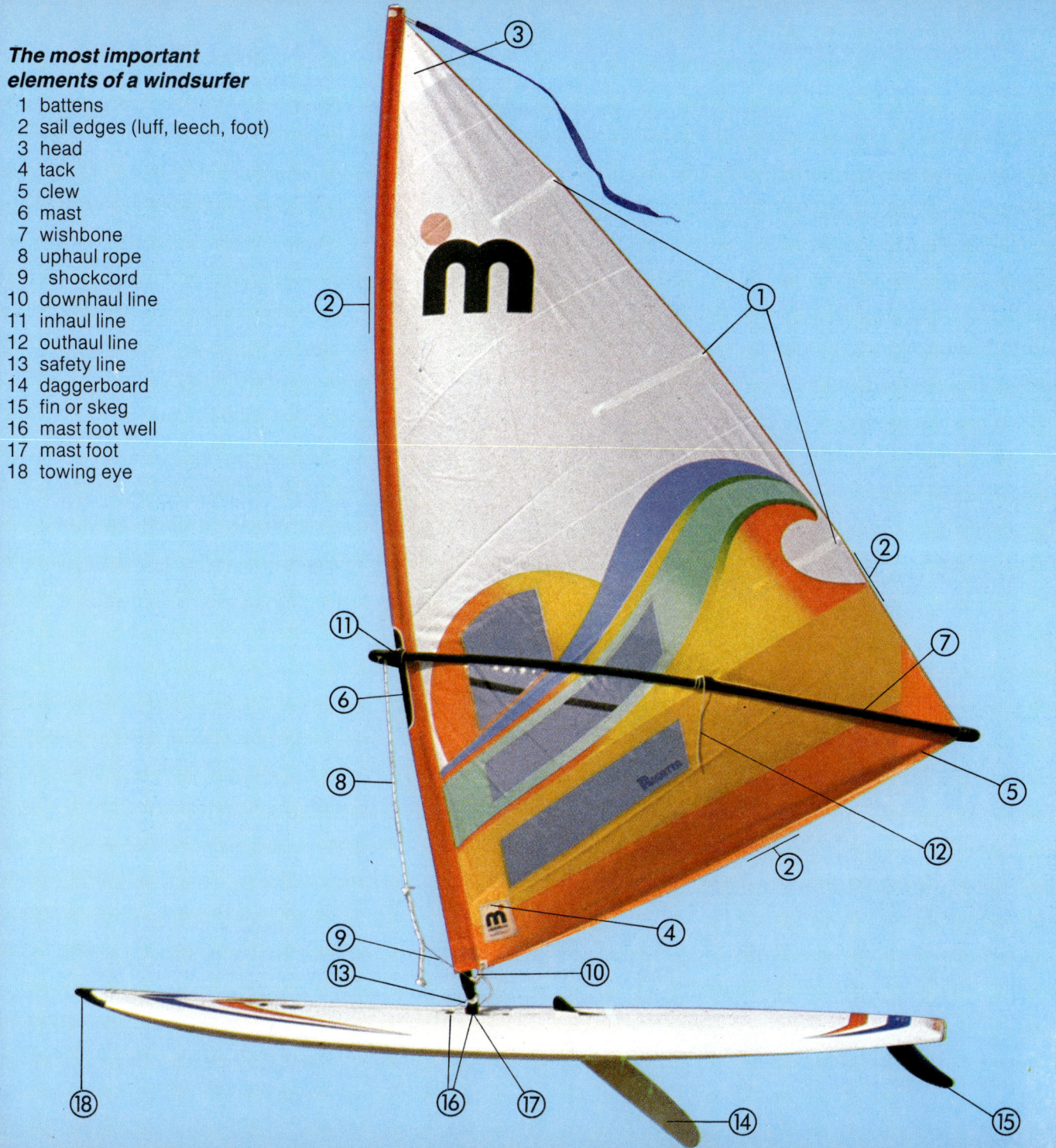

**The most important
elements of a windsurfer**

1 battens
2 sail edges (luff, leech, foot)
3 head
4 tack
5 clew
6 mast
7 wishbone
8 uphaul rope
9 shockcord
10 downhaul line
11 inhaul line
12 outhaul line
13 safety line
14 daggerboard
15 fin or skeg
16 mast foot well
17 mast foot
18 towing eye

Trim sail without creases

Having set up the sail, check whether there are still any creases in it. To do this, stand the sail up and point it towards the wind. The best idea is to examine the sail carefully from leeward, as it is easier to see creases from that direction. First, let the sail flap, and then sheet it in slowly. By following the seams between the cloths, you can see whether the belly of the sail is in the right place. When filled by the wind, the leeward side of the sail should not touch the wishbone. If you want to sail in breezy weather, trim the sail somewhat flatter (see illustration on page 14).

Now trim the sail, using the outhaul and downhaul lines in turn, until the sail is completely crease-free.

You won't be able to do this with every sail. If it is too old, or if it is not appropriate for the stiffness of your mast, you will just have to put up with a few small creases.

After some time on the water, you will find that you will often need to tauten the downhaul line somewhat, as the modern nylon material used for the mast sleeve always gives a little in the water.

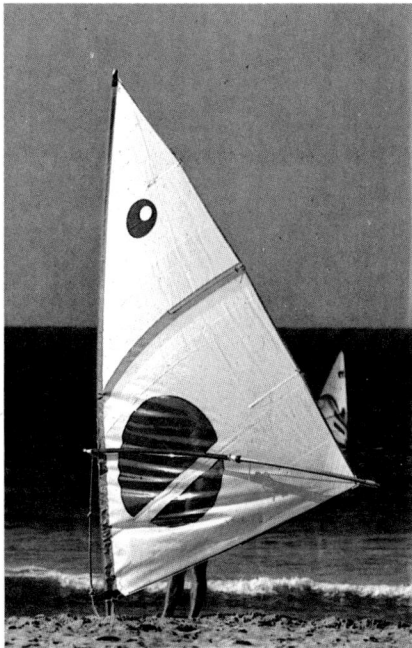

If the downhaul line has not been tautened sufficiently, it produces heavy creases from the mast across to the clew. Cure: tauten the downhaul line. As you do so, make sure that the mast sleeve is not pulled on to the inhaul line

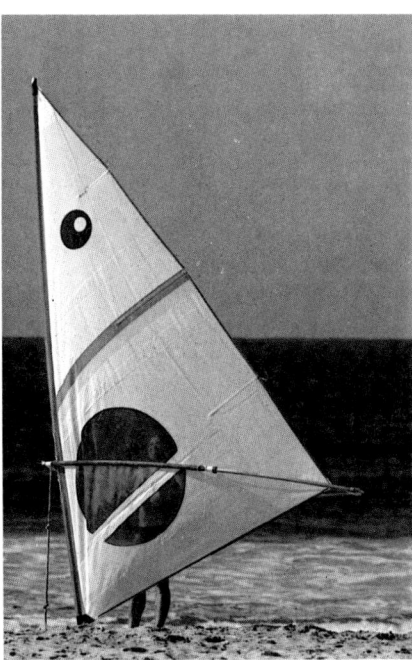

The creases running from top to bottom directly behind the mast are clearly visible. Cure: tauten the outhaul line

Carrying the board to the water

When you have finished checking your board and rig, carry them to the water one at a time. The following method is the one to use when

- the water is calm and there is not much of a wind, and/or
- you need to set off from an awkward stretch of the bank or shore (pebbles, jetties, etc.), where you cannot go for a beach start (see page 45), or
- when the beach is so blocked by other surfers and swimmers that you have to carry your equipment over or round them.

First, take the rig, with the mast at right angles to the wind, and with the sail to leeward, and pick it up by the mast. There are two methods of carrying it, and in both cases, you will be helped by the wind.

- With one hand, take hold of the wishbone from above, and with the other hand, take hold of the mast above the wishbone. Pick the rig up and carry it carefully to the water's edge, and put it down there. This method is advisable if the beach only slopes gently, or if there are strong gusts of wind, or if the wind keeps changing direction.
- Lift the sail over your head by the mast, and take hold of the wishbone from below with your other hand. Then you can carry the sail over your head and are more mobile than when you are holding it from above.

Whichever method you choose, however, watch out for other surfers and other beach-users, and bear in mind that until you are experienced, it will only take a gust of wind to send the rig flying round your ears — or someone else's!

It is therefore a good idea to find an open space to practise carrying the rig over your head. As long as you stand to windward with the sail to leeward, nothing can go wrong.

Next, carry the board to the water (with the daggerboard and skeg inserted). Put it down in water knee-deep. (Careful: if it is shallower, the skeg might break). Then paddle or walk to the rig and insert the mast foot. Do not forget to attach the safety line (see page 15).

On crowded beaches, to avoid disturbing other people, you should pack the rig up as you would when waiting to be rescued (see page 54), carry it right to the water's edge, and trim it there. Avoid flamboyant gestures like hurling the rig into the water. If there is a strong onshore wind, it might come flying back at you like a boomerang.

Getting the board and the rig out of the water

At the end of your surfing trip, go through the same procedure in reverse. After disconnecting the board and the rig, carry the board ashore first. Do not leave it right by the water, but carry it some distance back, to keep the shore clear. There is nothing more annoying than having to clamber over piles of other people's boards to reach the water. Then take the rig out of the water, and put it down some distance away from the water, with the mast at right angles to the wind, and the sail to leeward. Undo the outhaul line straight away, so that the rig does not fly away. If you want to take proper care of the sail, untie the downhaul line as well, and lay it down out of the wind.

Carrying the sail and the board. It is easier to carry two boards with someone else

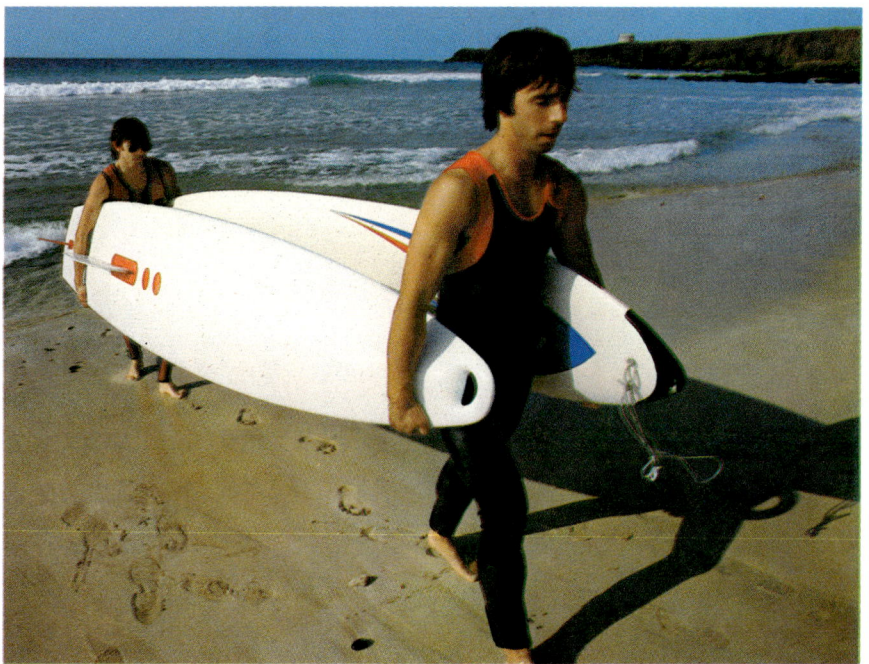

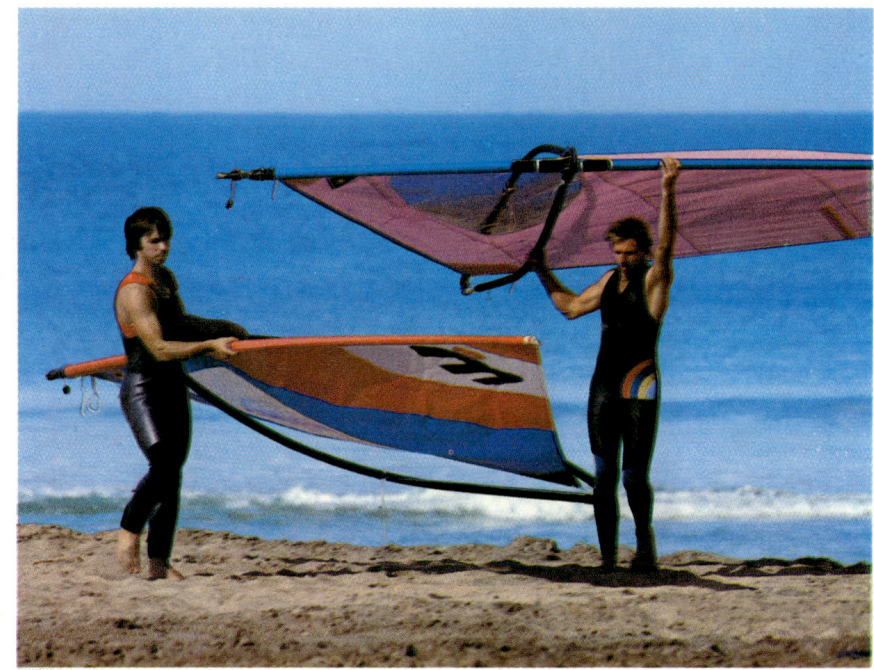

Pulling up the sail

Part of the fun in windsurfing is the occasional tumble into the water, and this is particularly likely to happen when you are continually working on improving your technique and trying out difficult manoeuvres. Pulling up the rig is a necessary part of the exercise, and an exhausting one, too. For this reason, it is necessary to make sure that your surfing fun lasts as long as possible, which means that you need a suitable rig and the right energy-saving technique. This will avoid straining your spine. Backache is the result of using the wrong technique.

The following tips will help you to save energy:
- choose a small sail with a short wishbone
- make sure that the uphaul rope reaches down to the mast foot
- make sure that you are standing properly
- always keep your back straight when pulling up the sail
- make use of your whole body-weight by leaning back slightly.

The sail is always pulled up from leeward. We describe the most suitable technique below. On page 20, you will find out how to bring the sail round from windward to leeward.

1

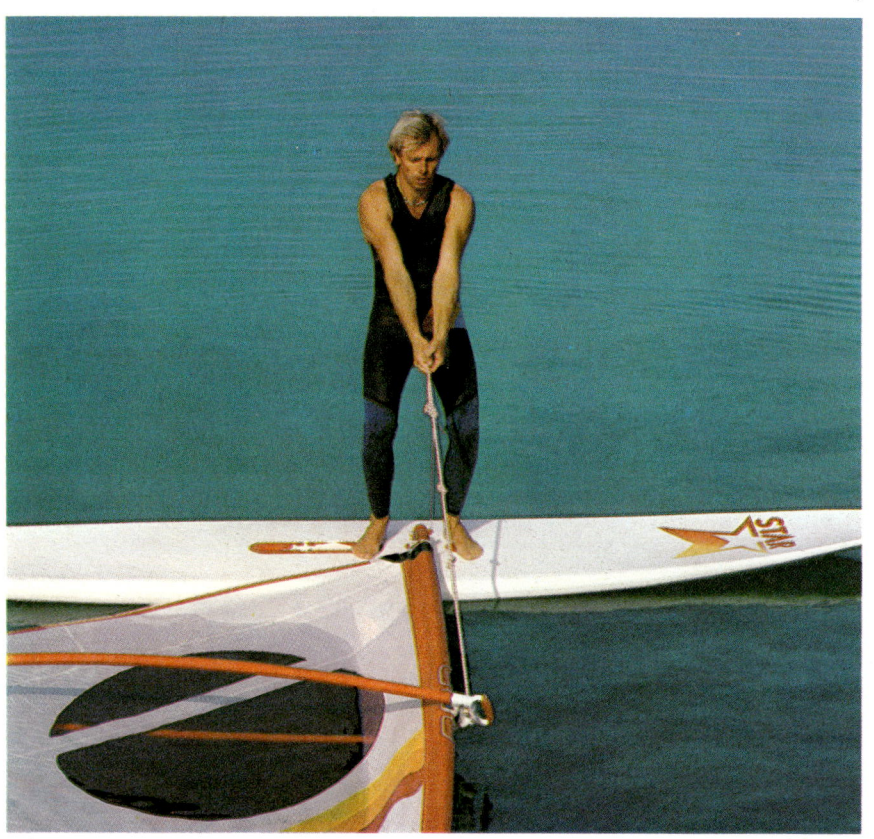

● Place your feet a hand's breadth to the left and right of the mast

You can of course have your feet closer together or farther apart. What is important, however, is that you should place both feet *the same distance* from the mast, and that you balance your weight *equally* on both feet. Otherwise, you would unintentionally make the board turn round.

● Have the mast exactly abeam (at 90° to the board)

Standing on the board, pull gently sideways on the uphaul rope to change the position of the board relative to the rig, until the mast is exactly abeam of the board. Only in this way can you avoid having to pull crookedly on the uphaul rope (illustration 1).

● Starting position

The rig lies to leeward. the mast exactly abeam. Stand with your feet a hand's breadth to the left and right of the mast foot, with your toes pointing to the mast tip. Take hold of the uphaul line by the lowest knot, bend your knees slightly, and straighten your back. Keep your head up (illustration 2).

● Stretch your legs — pull the mast out of the water

Keep your shoulders leaning back slightly and straighten your legs. Keep your back and your arms straight. In this way, you will pull the mast up out of the water. You will then feel that the resistance is noticeably reduced: the water drains out of the mast sleeve and off part of the sail. Wait until all the water has drained off before continuing (illustration 3).

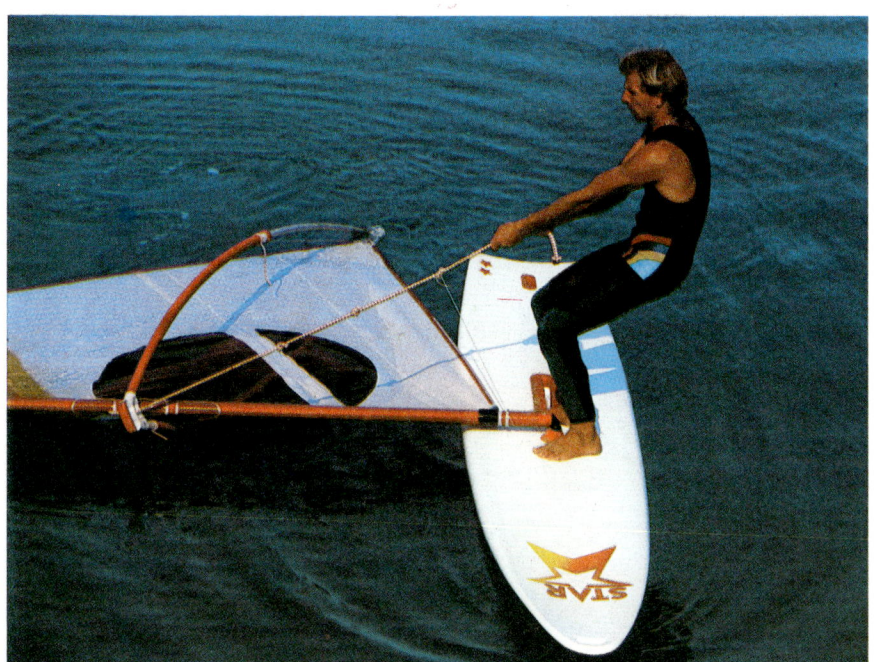

● **Pull the rig completely out of the water**

Pull the sail up hand over hand, until it is completely out of the water. Keep your back straight.

● **Take hold of the mast and assume the basic position**

Take hold of the mast with one or both hands. Keep your arms stretched out. In this way, you can stand steadily and keep your balance better. The end of the wishbone must not touch the water. Stand with your knees relaxed, look up, and remain at right angles to the rig and the board. You are now standing in the *basic position* (see illustration below).

▲ 2   ▼ 3

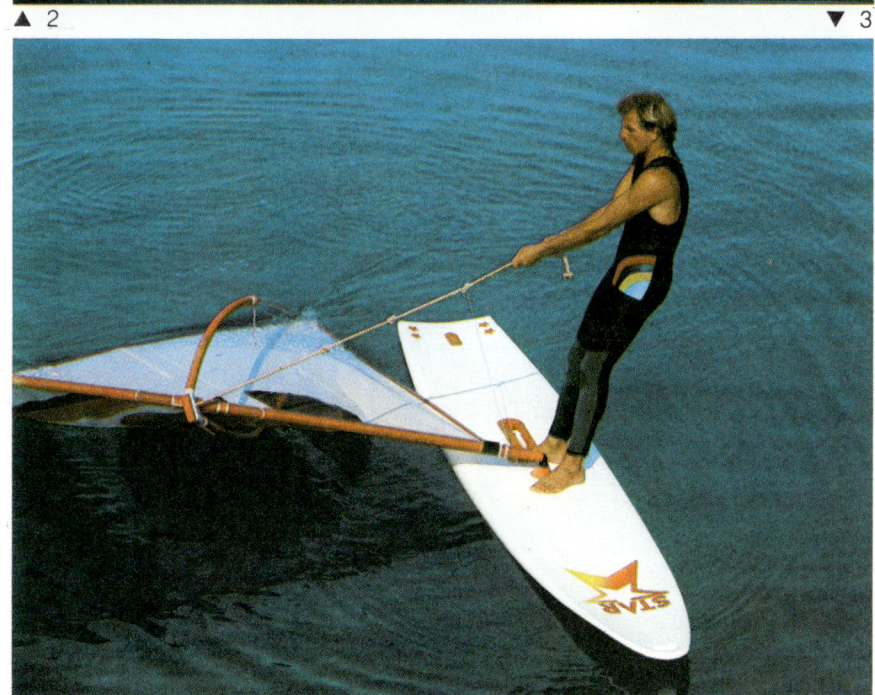

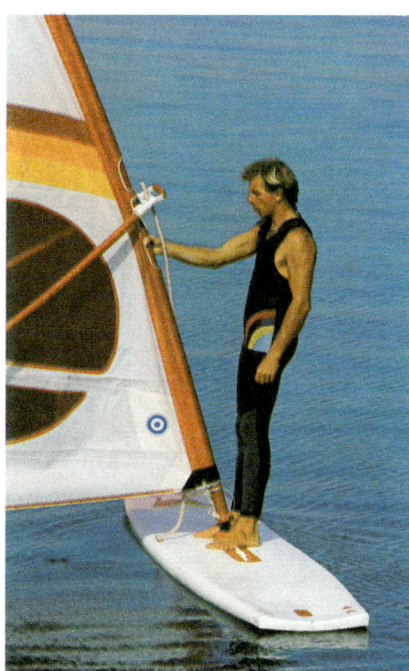

Bringing the rig round from windward to leeward

When you sit down on your board for a short rest on the water, it will hardly take a minute and you will find that the rig is floating on the windward side of the board. The wind resistance of your body and the board have made you drift round your rig to leeward. Falling off to windward is another thing that can make you have to bring your rig round to leeward before actually pulling up the sail.

There are two techniques you can use for this, depending on whether you want to carry on in the same direction or to turn your board round.

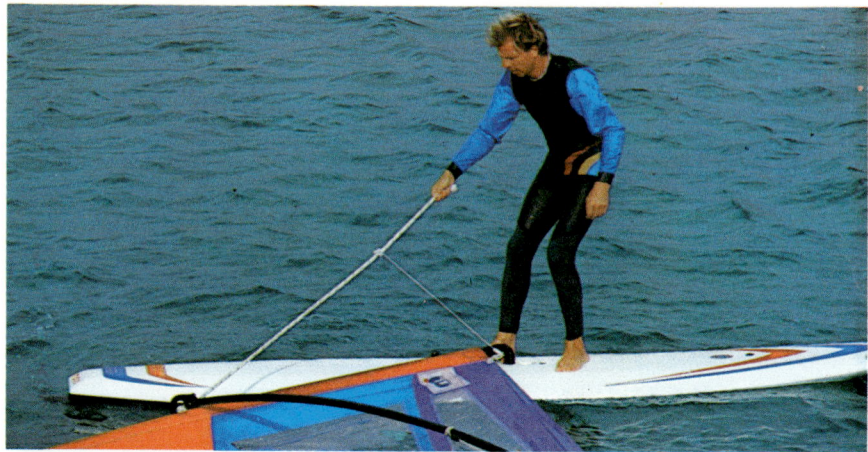

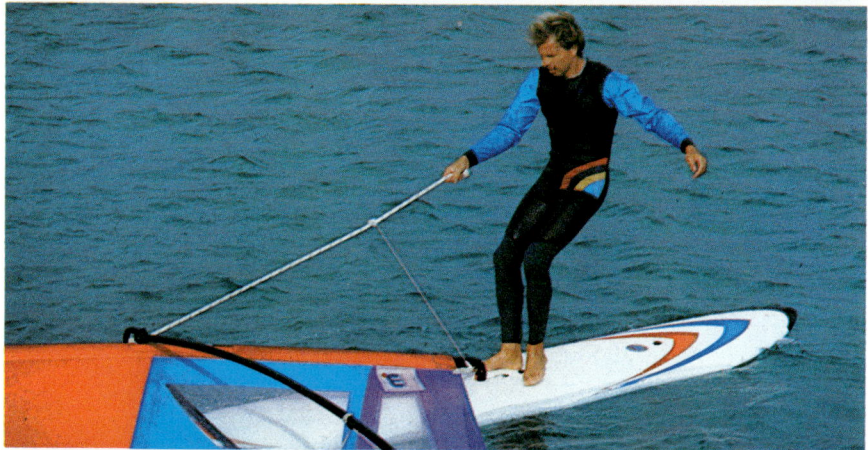

If you want to carry on in the same direction:

lift the rig by the uphaul line and pull it over the bow or stern. Keep your toes pointing at the mast top. When the rig is lying on top of the board, you will have an unsteady moment to overcome. Carry on pulling quickly, until the rig is once again lying completely in the water to leeward, with the mast abeam.

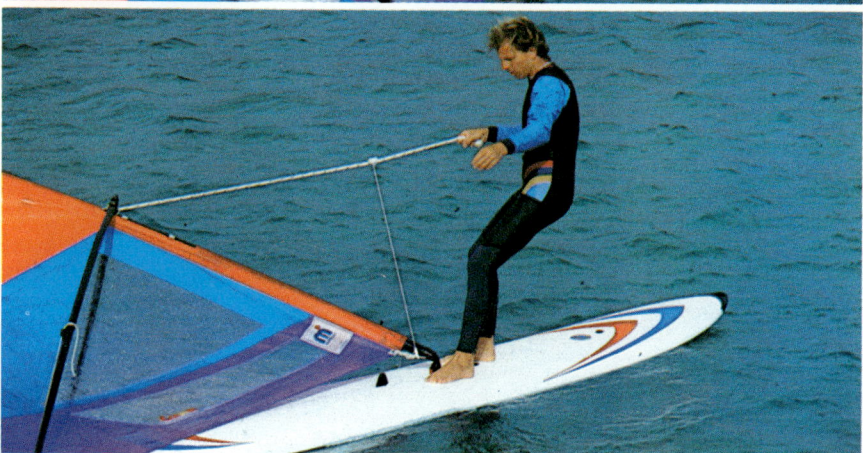

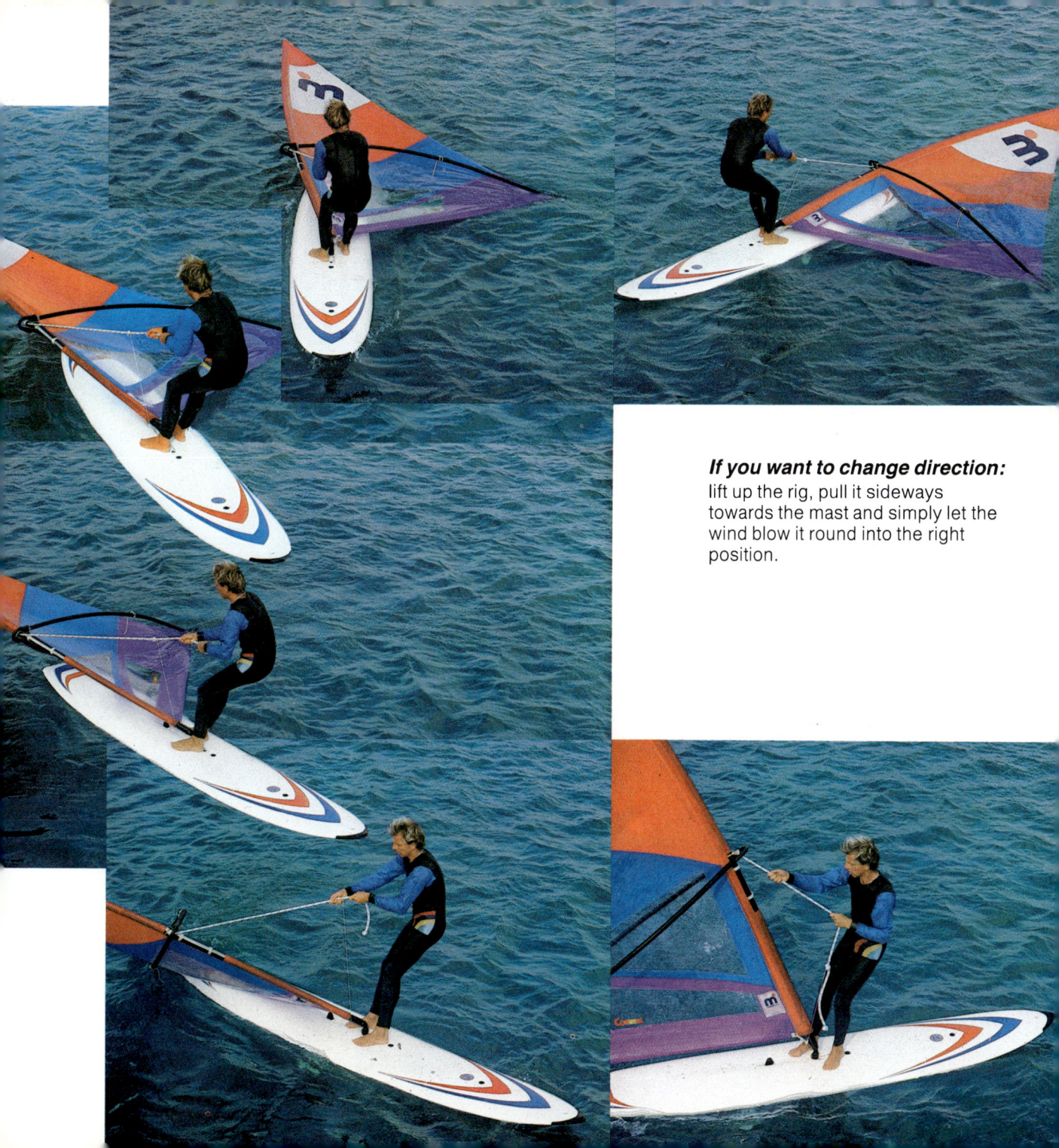

If you want to change direction: lift up the rig, pull it sideways towards the mast and simply let the wind blow it round into the right position.

Half turn

The simplest method of reversing the sail is to begin in the basic position and incline the rig into the wind, in the direction of the bow or stern. You will need this technique again and again, whenever you need to set your board at right angles to the wind, and also to manoeuvre yourself out of a tight situation.

Begin in the basic position. Take hold of the mast with one hand only; then you will be standing firmly. Start by quickly raking the sail fore and aft. Use your mast hand to rake the rig towards the bow, and the sheet hand to rake it towards the stern. In each case, the end of the board towards which you are pointing the rig will bear away from the wind. If you want to reverse the sail, i.e. to turn the board round 180°, keep the rig inclined into the

wind and raked in one direction until the board has made a half turn under your feet.

In making a half turn, pay particular attention to the following:

● Keep your arm stretched just far enough, so that the end of the wishbone is only a couple of inches above the surface of the water. Like this, the board will turn quickest, and you will be standing most firmly.

● When you move your feet, always keep your toes pointing at the end of the wishbone.

● Keep your steps as small as possible, and always stand over the middle of the board.

Exercise:

By making a few half turns, over the stern in each case, try to sail a short distance against the wind. This should be quite easy if you make the turns carefully.

Getting under way
Basic position

In order to set off under ideal conditions, arrange the rig at right angles to the board. The rig serves as a type of weather vane, with the end of the wishbone pointing to leeward. Now you can take your time to have a look round and get your bearings. Make use of the time in the basic position to check the following details, depending on your skill and what is going on around you (see illustration below):

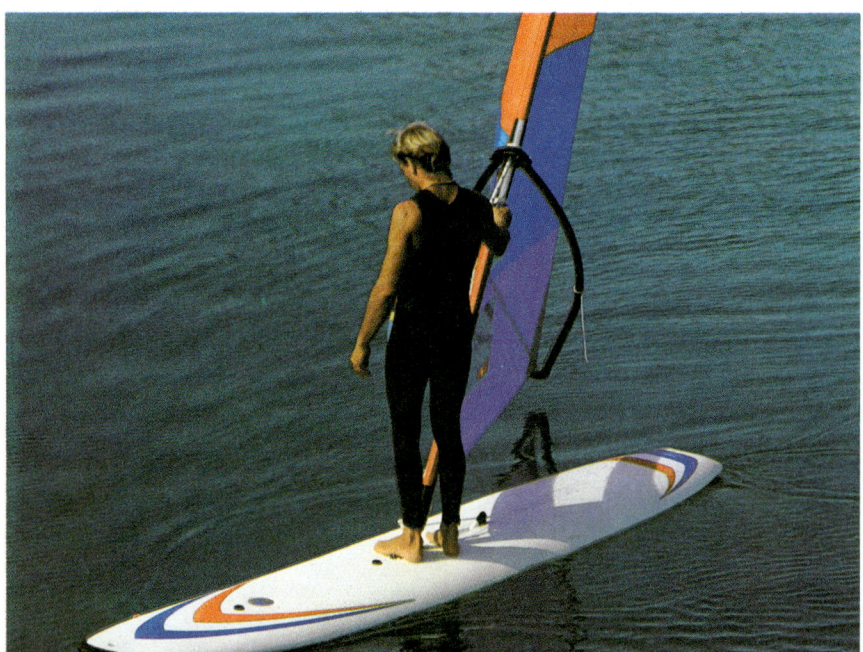

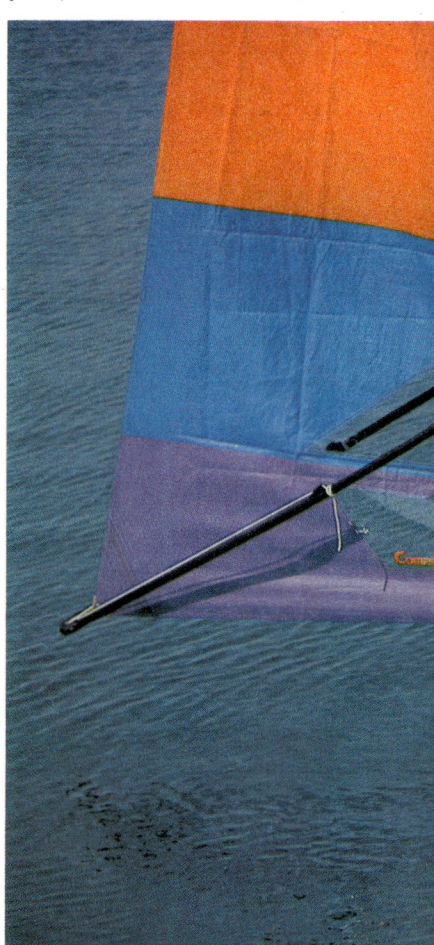

- Which direction is my bow pointing in?
- What point shall I be aiming at when reaching?
- Are there any swimmers or divers around?
- Are there any currents to make me drift?
- Are there any other surfers directly in front of my bow?
- How far away from my starting point am I?

Checking the amount of space available

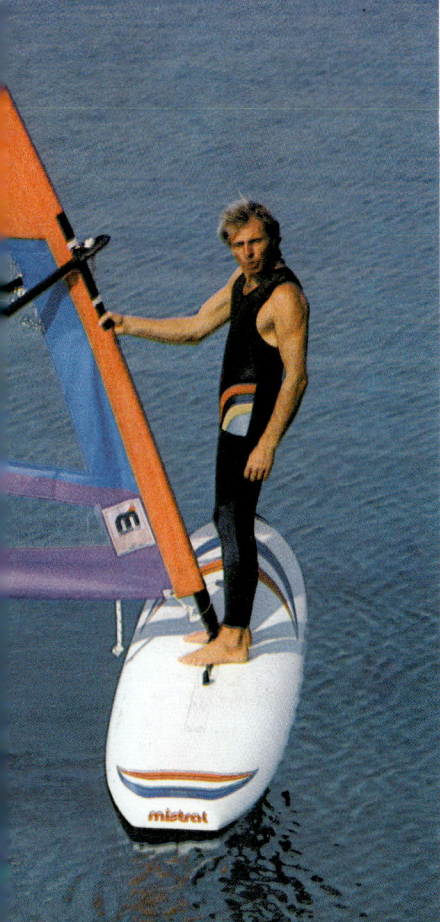

Starting position

Particularly as a beginner, you should make sure that you adopt the correct starting position. The following movements will bring you into the starting position:

- let go of the mast with what will become your sheet hand
- place your rear foot some distance behind the mast
- place your front foot just behind the mast
- keep your feet parallel and as close as possible to the midship line.
- keep your toes pointing diagonally forward.
- keep your arm holding the mast as straight as possible.

In the case of an experienced surfer, the starting position and the basic position will tend more and more to coincide, which means that at this point, as in the basic position, you should pause and look round for a moment.

Different positions for your feet

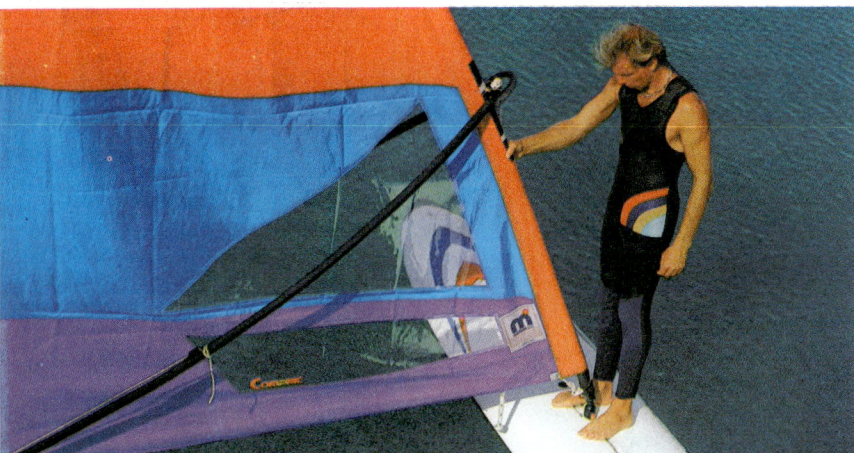

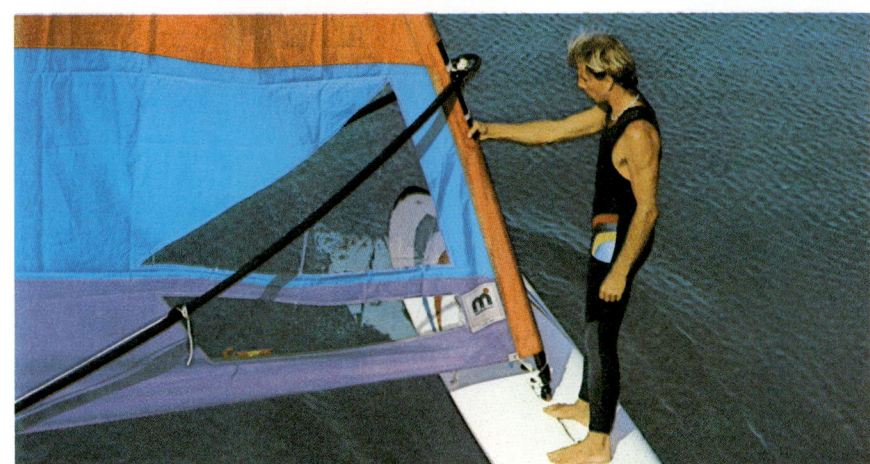

Getting under way

The first series of photographs on these two pages is intended to give an overall view of how to get under way. The second series shows the same process in detail.

Experience has shown that it is with this manoeuvre, which is the first one for the beginner, that most mistakes occur. Very often, he does not place his feet far enough behind the mast foot, and above all he does not pull the rig far enough round to windward.

The harder the wind is blowing, the further behind the mast foot you should place your feet, and the further to windward you should pull the rig.

Exercise:

The stop/go exercise is particularly good for learning how to master this difficult part of getting under way.

Simply move your shoulders back and forth, one after the other. As soon as you move your shoulders forwards again, the sail will flap and the board will lose headway. When you turn the upper part of your body back, the board will pick up speed again.

This exercise gives you a good feeling for how to handle the rig and makes it clear that you do not just sheet the sail in with your after hand, but that sheeting in and out are actions for which you should always use the whole of the upper part of your body. It is important to know this when it comes to surfing in strong winds and using a harness.

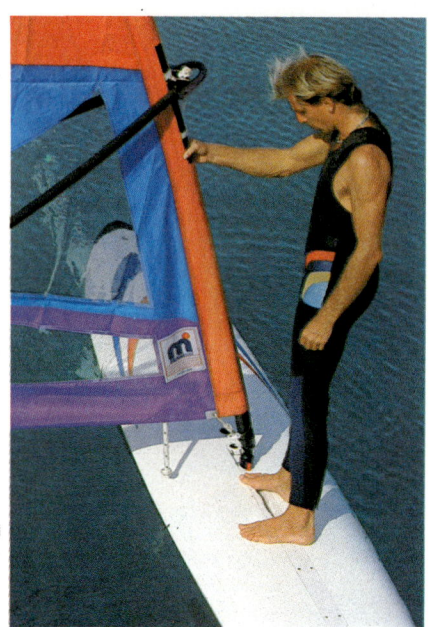

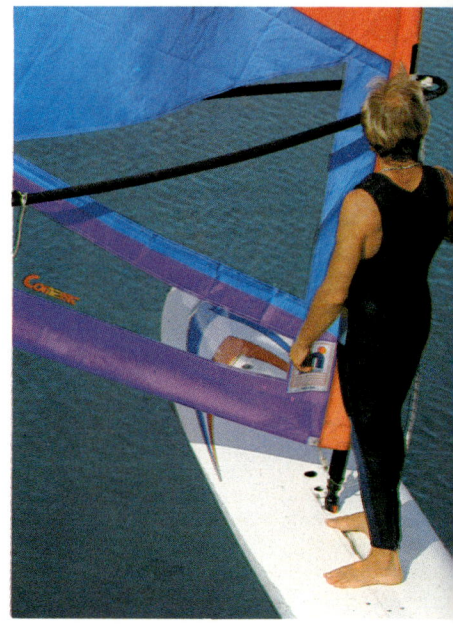

Remain in the starting position until you have made sure that the way ahead is clear, and that your board is at exactly 90° to the rig. Just as in the basic position, you can get your board pointing in the right direction by inclining the rig into the wind.

By turning the top part of your body, pull the rig *to windward* until it becomes quite light. Have a look through the window in the sail to make sure that your bow is still pointing at whatever target you want to get to when reaching.

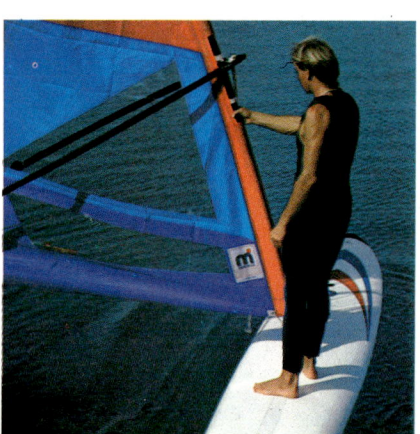

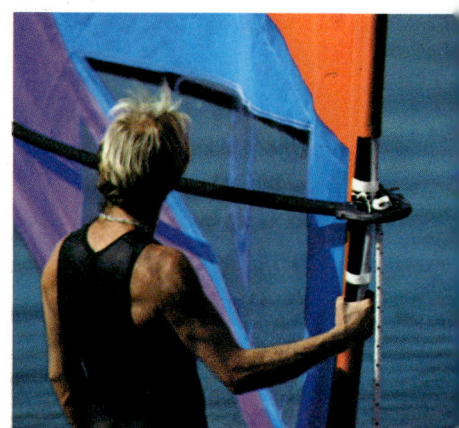

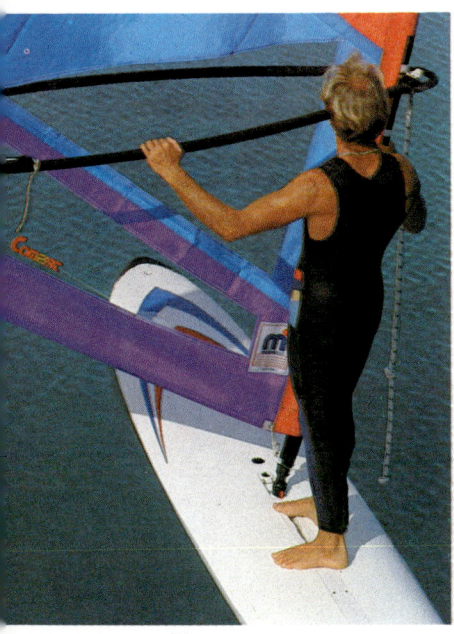

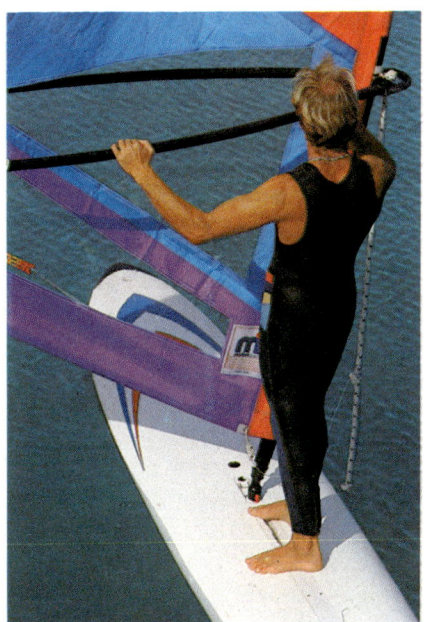

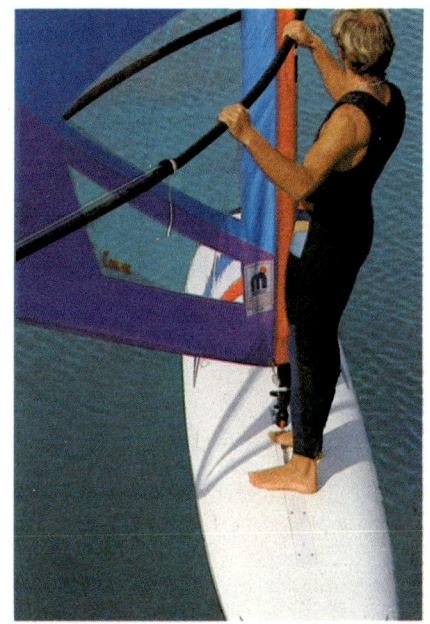

Place your *sheet hand* gently on the wishbone. If you keep your thumb on top, too, you will reduce the strain on your forearm. Note the position of the left hand in relation to the shoulder. Be careful that you are not accidentally sheeting in with your sheet hand.

Place your *mast hand* on the wishbone. You should now be resting both hands on the wishbone, about the width of your shoulders apart, and with the axis of your shoulders at right angles to the board. Now have one last check that you have got the board and sail at right angles to one another, and that you are pointing in the right direction

By turning your shoulders back, *sheet in* the sail just so far that it stops flapping. At the same time, lean back slightly and place your weight on your rear foot. Look ahead at the point you want to sail to. Keep your arms bent, with your elbows down.

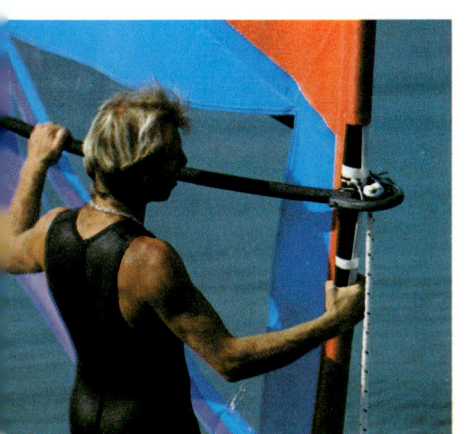

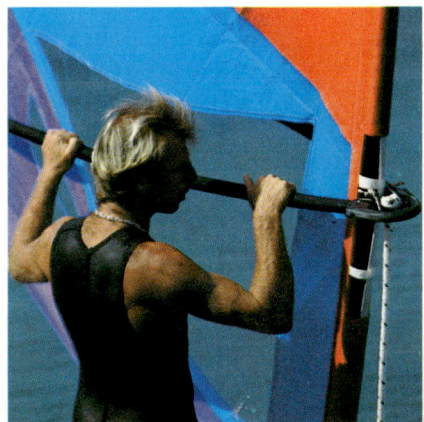

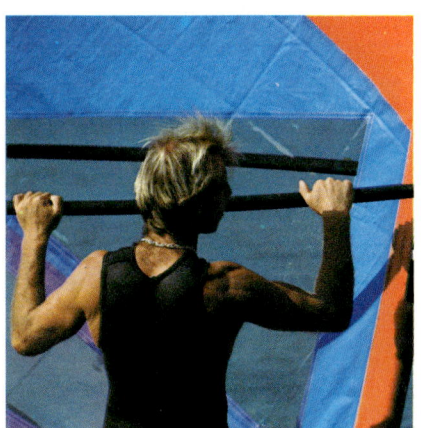

Emergency stops

Stopping quickly when you are sailing at full speed is a technique that you need to master perfectly. All too often, situations occur in which you can no longer take evasive action, but have to stop immediately. You are sailing behind a friend and he falls into the water because he has failed to anticipate a gust of wind; or a beginner who ought to keep to his course suddenly turns and sails into your path; or at the last minute you catch sight of a surfacing swimmer. In such a situation, you could of course simply let go of everything and jump into the water next to your board for good measure. The only trouble is

that to do this, you need plenty of room to leeward, otherwise your mast will fall on whatever it was you wanted to avoid.

For this purpose, the emergency stop is more suitable. It has the advantage that you keep your board under control, can get under way again immediately, and do not have the bother of pulling up the sail again.

To make an emergency stop,
turn the upper part of your body and press the sail firmly against the wind.

If you learn and practise the emergency stop in the following steps, you will be able to bring your board to a standstill in less than ten feet, even when you are sailing at full speed in a strong wind.

Exercises:
● Practise sheeting in and out alternately when reaching (stop/go) by turning the upper part of your body (see page 24).
● Sheet so far that your sail catches the wind from the "wrong side".
● Sheet out, and then press the rig hard against the wind.
● Practise under different conditions until you can feel the exact point you have to press against; then you can use the whole of your body-weight, and you will come to a halt immediately.
The emergency stop does not work, of course, when you are running, and it is very difficult when you are broad reaching. On these courses, you must take evasive action, because if you let go of your rig, it will fall in the direction you are sailing in and might hit the obstacle in your way.

The emergency gybe
This manoeuvre is necessary if you have to veer off in a very tight space after an emergency stop. To do this, keep the sail to starboard after the emergency stop. A tip: lower the clew (see illustration below) right down, and the board will turn quickly.

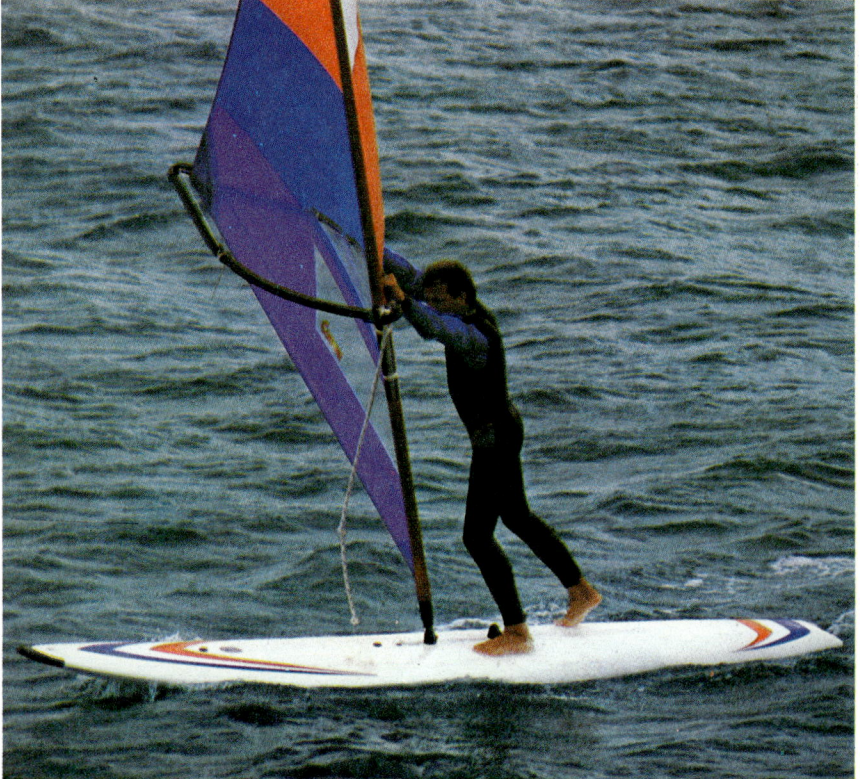

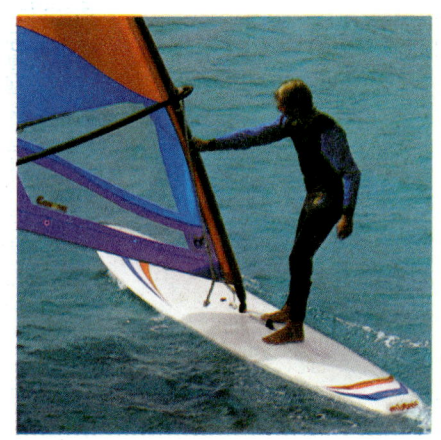

Steering

Surfboards are steered by tilting the rig along the chord of the sail and by tilting the board round its longitudinal axis (by putting weight on the edge of the board).

The most important requirement for steering properly is knowing the right position of the sail. On all upwind courses (see page 71), there is always only one correct position for the sail, which one finds when the sail *just stops flapping*.

In windsurfing, any change in direction is described with reference to the wind. You can change direction more towards the wind (heading up), or more away from the wind (bearing off) (see page 71).

● *To head up*, tilt *the rig to leeward in the plane of the sail,*
● *to bear off*, tilt *the rig to windward in the plane of the sail.*

At first it is important to keep the position of the sail in relation to the wind unchanged. Only when your board reacts by changing direction

daggerboards, the degree of the turn is increased by putting weight on the outer edge (i.e. the edge on the outside of the turn). If no daggerboard is fitted, the opposite is the case. Here, you increase the degree of the turn by putting your weight on the inner edge (i.e. the edge on the inside of the turn).

With all manoeuvres that require this kind of steering, we have proceeded on the assumption that we are dealing with boards fitted with daggerboards.

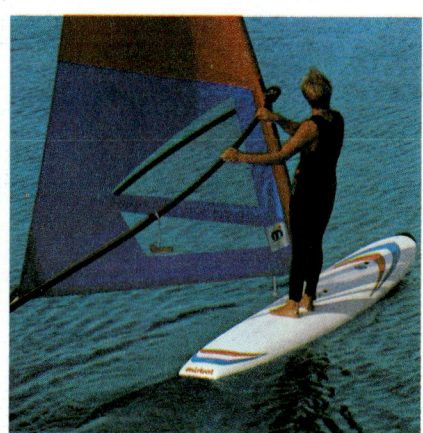

Heading up: tilt the rig to leeward in the plane of the sail

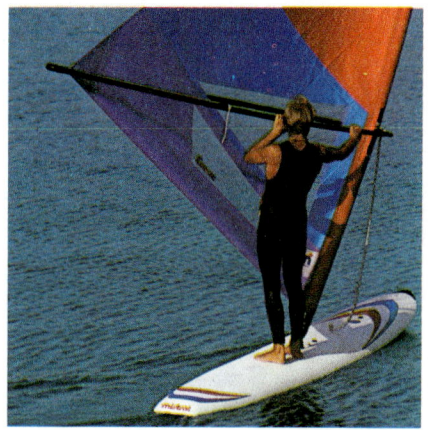

Bearing off: tilt the rig to windward in the plane of the sail

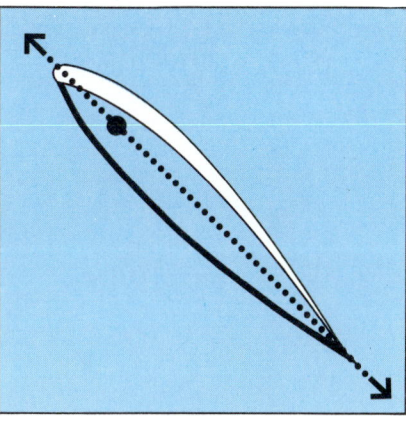

To steer, move the rig to leeward or windward in the plane of the sail

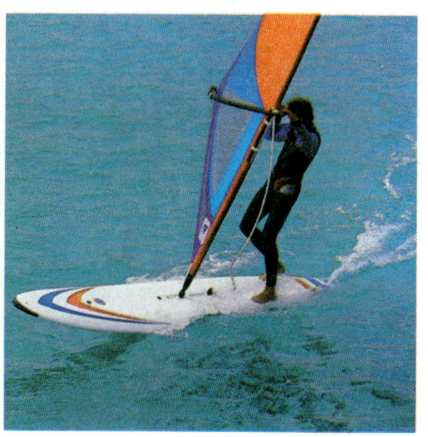

do you gradually adapt the position of your sail to the new direction. Whether you have your weight more on the front or the back foot during this process is of no importance as far as steering is concerned.

Foot steering works differently. If you tilt the board sideways by putting your weight on the edge, you will either increase or reduce the change in direction caused by tilting the rig.

In the case of boards fitted with

To bear off, put your weight on the outer edge

Heading up
Tilting the rig to leeward in the plane of the sail, without changing the position of the sail at first (or: "clew down"). Put your weight on the leeward edge of the board.

Bearing off
Tilting the rig to windward in the plane of the sail, without changing the position of the sail at first (or: "clew up"). Put your weight on the windward edge of the board.

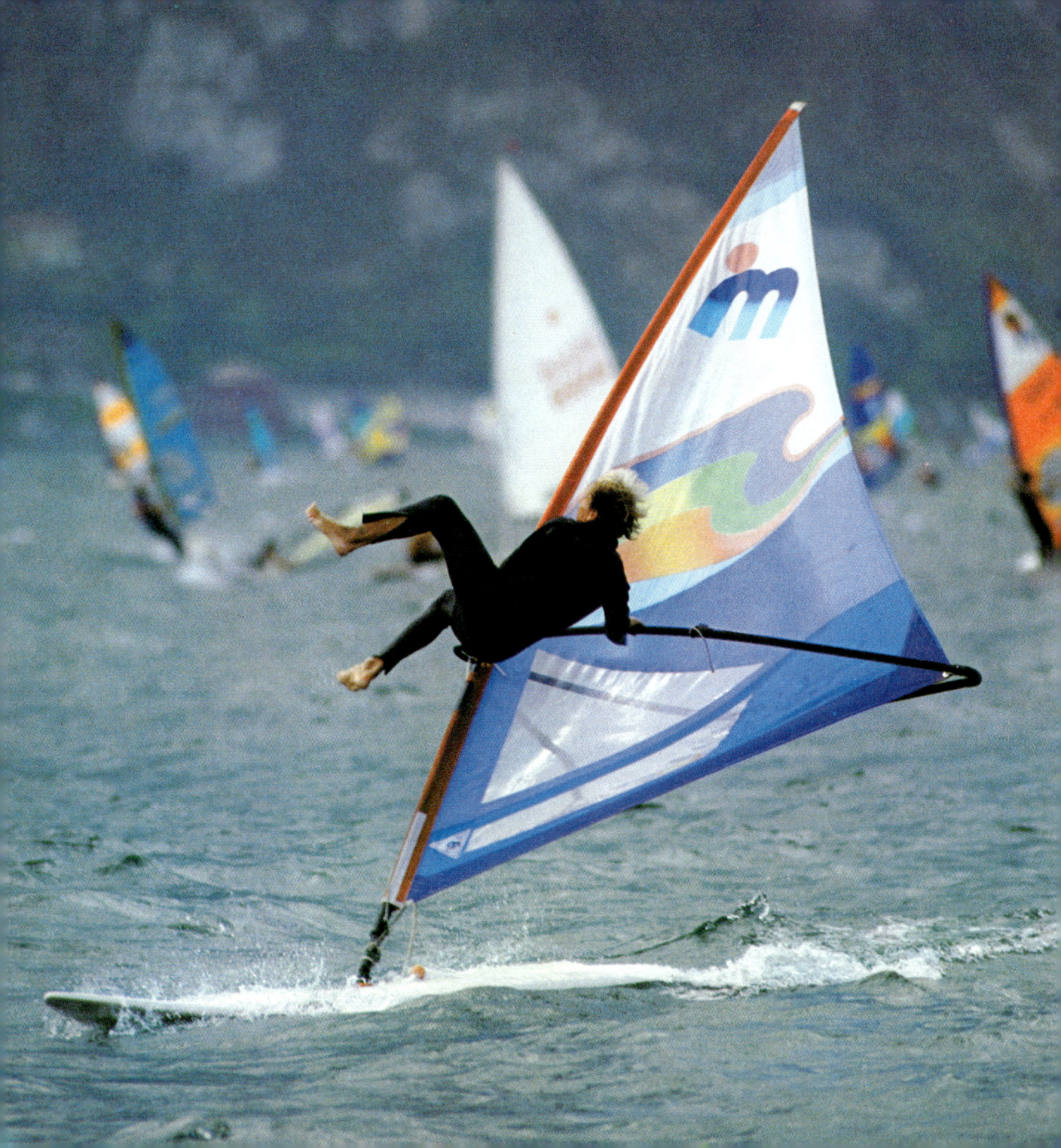

When several mistakes in steering are made, the result is often a *catapult fall*. At first, you will not be able to manage such a spectacular performance as is demonstrated here, but if you make all the following mistakes at the same time, you will be well on the way to it. If you

● try to bear off by placing your front foot in front of the mast and "pushing the board out of the wind",
● and bend your hips forwards as you do so,
● and sheet the sail in far beyond the correct sail position,

then the rig ought really to send you flying forwards. If you do not take off, then the only explanation is that you must have got your feet fixed in the footstraps or stuck in the daggerboard case.

But joking apart, to avoid unintentional catapult falls, and to practise precise steering, we have worked out a few exercises for you, because it is in steering that a number of typical mistakes are made again and again — and not only by beginners — which could be straightened out by means of a few simple exercises.

Exercises

● Keep your feet close together and alternately head up and bear off by tilting the rig exactly along the plane of the sail.
● Steer with both feet *in front of* the mast foot.
● Steer with both feet *behind* the daggerboard case.
● When reaching, practise walking up and down the board a little. If you only change your position as you do so, but do not alter the position of the sail, your board will carry on sailing straight ahead.

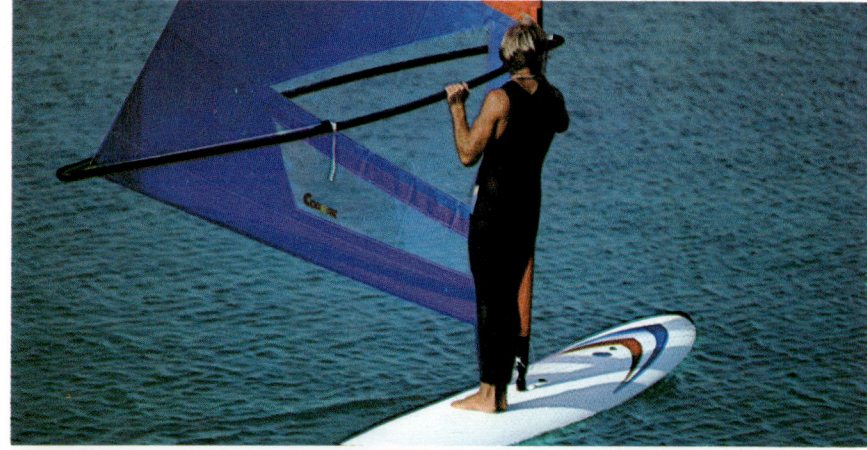

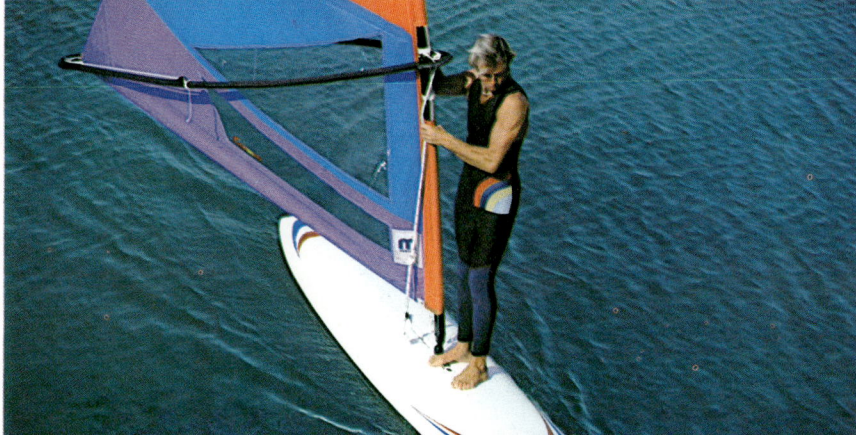

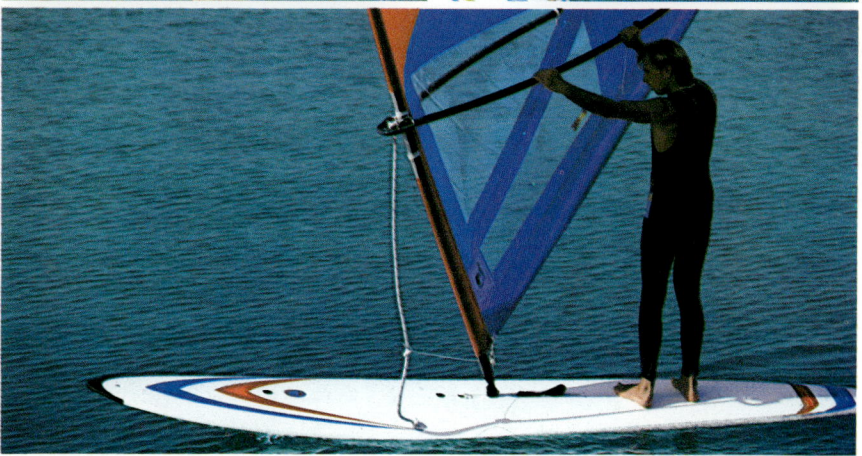

Turning

On these two pages, we have demonstrated two different ways of turning. You will see that the variant intended for strong winds, or "fast turn", is not only carried out much more quickly, but also leaves out part of the basic beginner's turn.

The individual stages of the beginner's turn

- Head up until beating
- Place mast hand on mast
- Place front foot by mast
- Head up until heading to wind, let go with sail hand, and step in front of mast
- Change hands on mast
- Carry on turning by inclining the sail into the wind, until you are back in the basic position
- Move off again

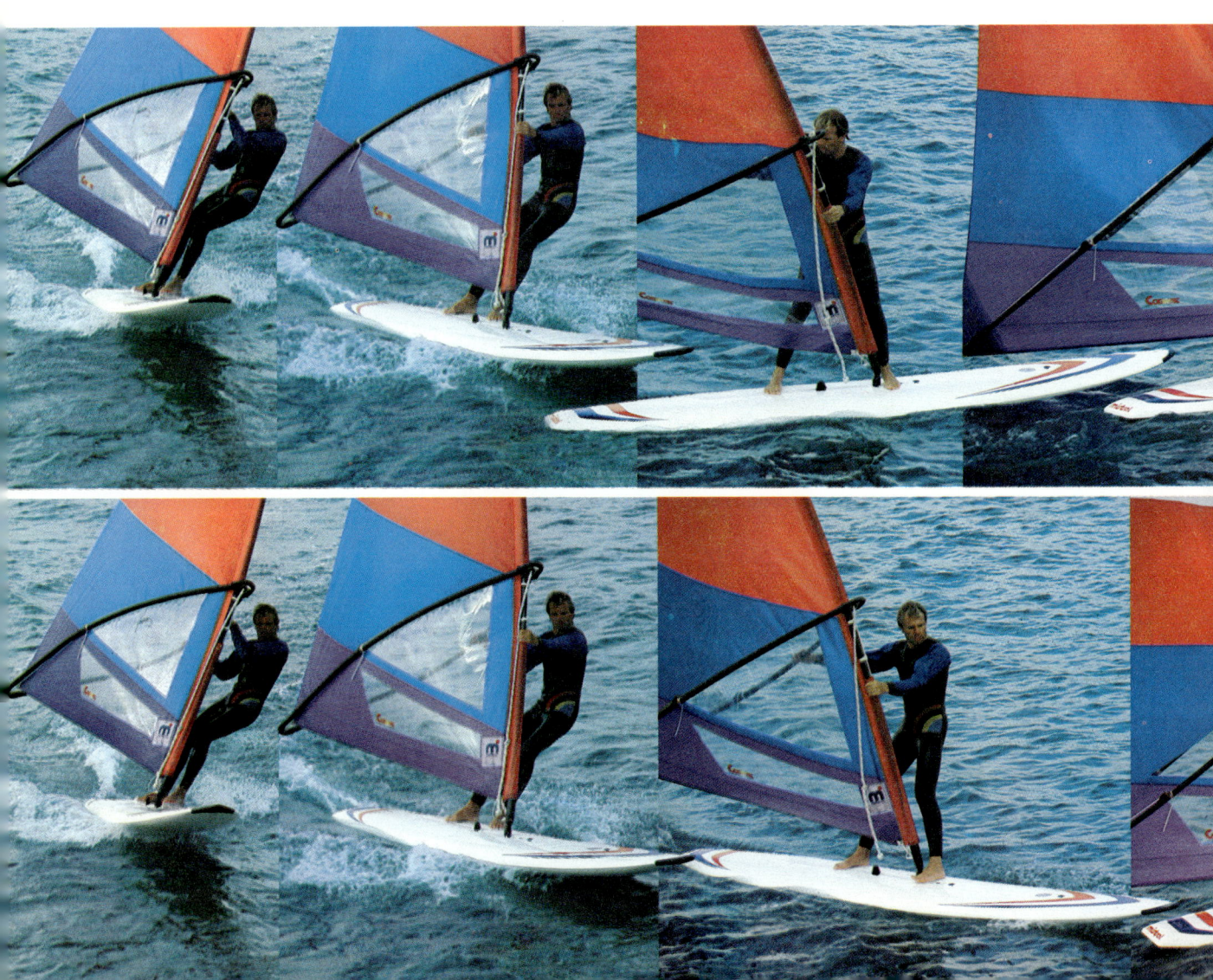

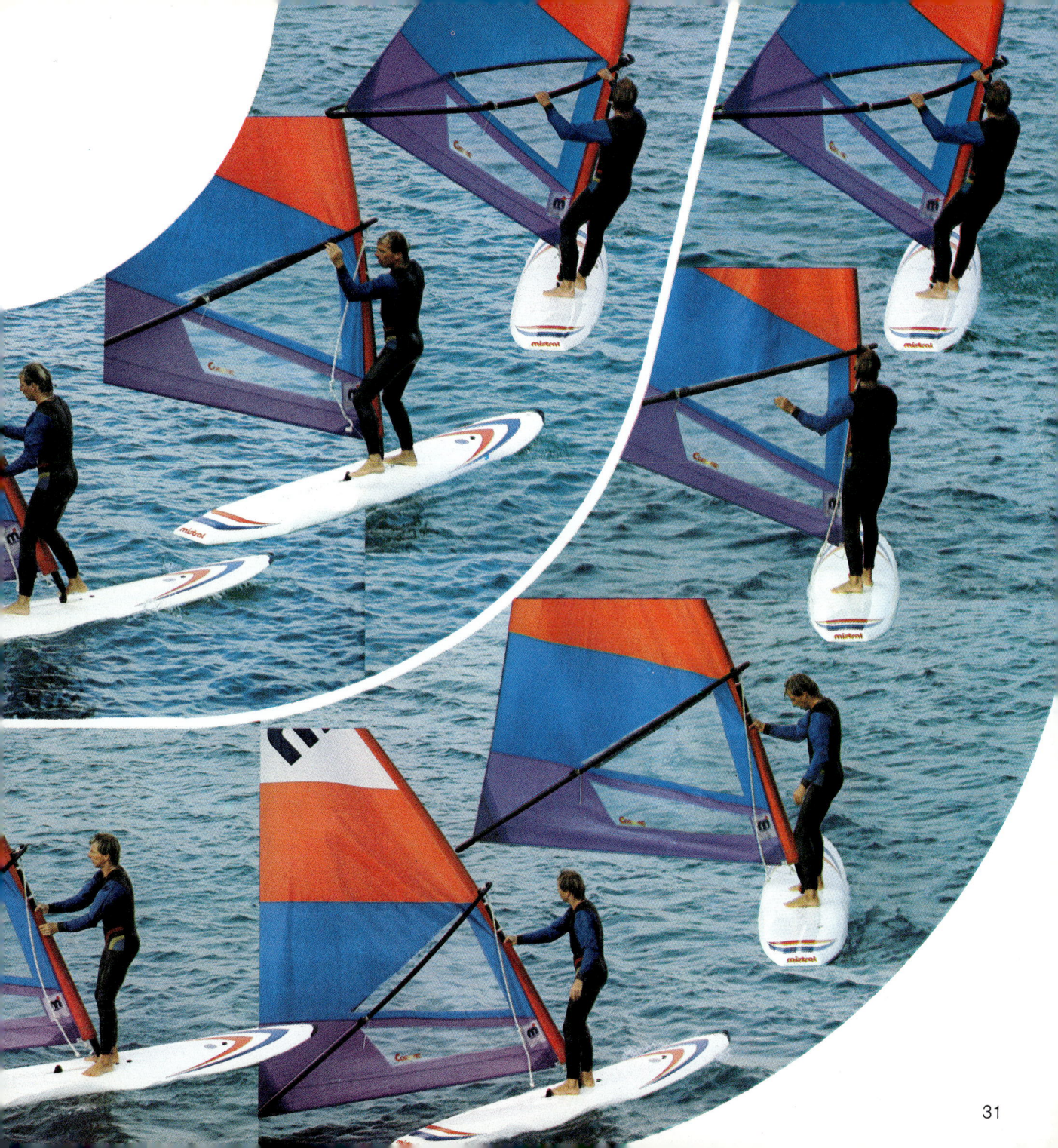

For a fast turn, you need to:
- turn the board by heading up quickly until it just passes through the eye of the wind,
- turn on the ball of your front foot,
- move your back foot up to your front foot,
- let go of the mast with your former mast hand and take hold of it with your new mast hand,
- pull the mast to windward and at the same time take a step towards the stern, and
- move off on a beat straight away.

The fast turn has two aims, both of which need to be achieved:
- *moving to the opposite side of the sail as quickly and as safely as possible*
- *gaining as much distance as possible against the wind.*

It will only be possible to achieve these two aims if:
- you head up carefully and always keep the sail in the ideal position
- you begin to move round the sail at exactly the right moment and carry out the manoeuvre firmly and crisply.

The photographs below demonstrate the most important stages of the fast turn, once again with close-ups of the grip technique and the foot positions. The first photograph in each case shows the initial position, the second shows the moment at which you actually change sides over the bow, and the

third shows the preparation for moving off again.

As you can see, it is not a big step from the beginner's turn to the fast turn.

In fact, it is only the second half of the fast turn that is slightly different, since in the case of the beginner's turn, this includes the somewhat complicated "half turn", whereas with the advanced version, you move off again immediately.

One thing is important if you want to learn and master the fast turn in such a way that you can carry it out as a smooth manoeuvre: begin by practising the movements in slow motion, making them as "gentle" as possible. If you then increase the

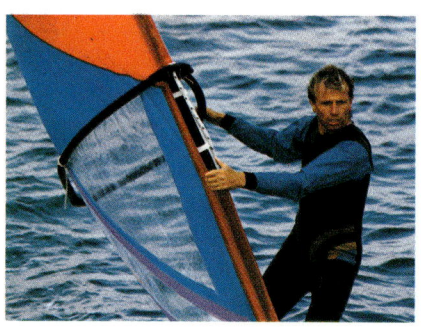

With your mast hand on the mast, head up until the board passes through the eye of the wind

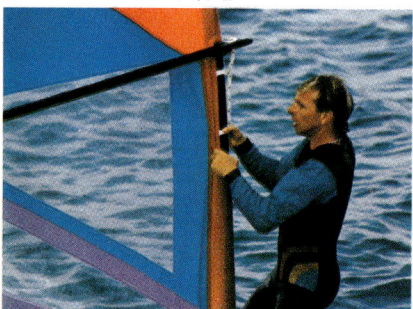

Transfer your sheet hand to the mast, let go with your former mast hand, keep the mast close to your body

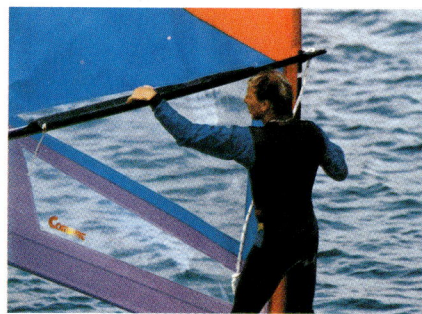

Pull the mast to windward with your new mast hand and move off again immediately

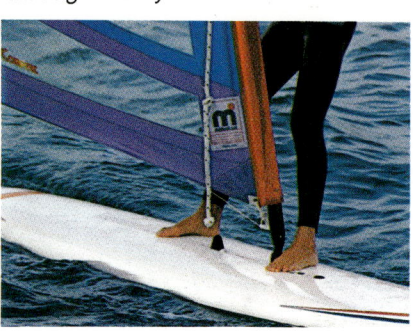

While reaching, place your front foot immediately in front of the mast

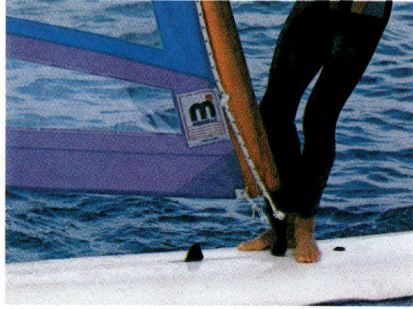

Turn on the ball of your foot and move your rear foot up to it

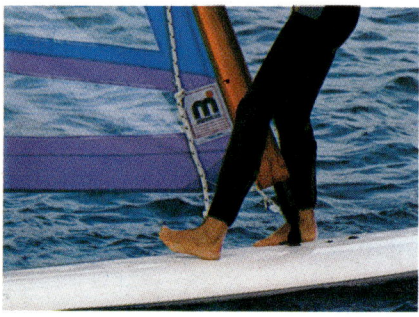

Continue turning on the ball of your rear foot, and step towards the stern

speed gradually, the turn will remain smooth, and you will not develop any bad habits, such as jumping hectically round the mast.

The following exercises will help you:

Exercises

- Carry out a series of turns, one after the other, always leaving one hand on the mast.
- Move off on a reach from the initial position.
- Head up until you are heading into the wind, and bear off immediately.
- If you want to practise the movements especially carefully, simply lay your board flat on the ground, after removing the daggerboard and skeg — the best idea is to find a flat piece of grass or a stretch of soft sand. Lay it down in such a way that the tip of the board is pointing almost directly into the wind. Now stand on the "old" windward side, which is already pointing slightly to leeward, as though you had just headed up and passed through the eye of the wind. With this exercise, you eliminate the movement of the board and can concentrate completely on moving to the other side of the sail. When you have got your front foot in front of the mast and your front hand (mast hand) on the mast, you are standing correctly.

Practise the following three stages:

- stepping in front of the mast and changing hands
- stepping well back and at the same time pulling the mast hard forwards and to windward
- moving off on a reach with your hand on the mast.

Concentration while heading up

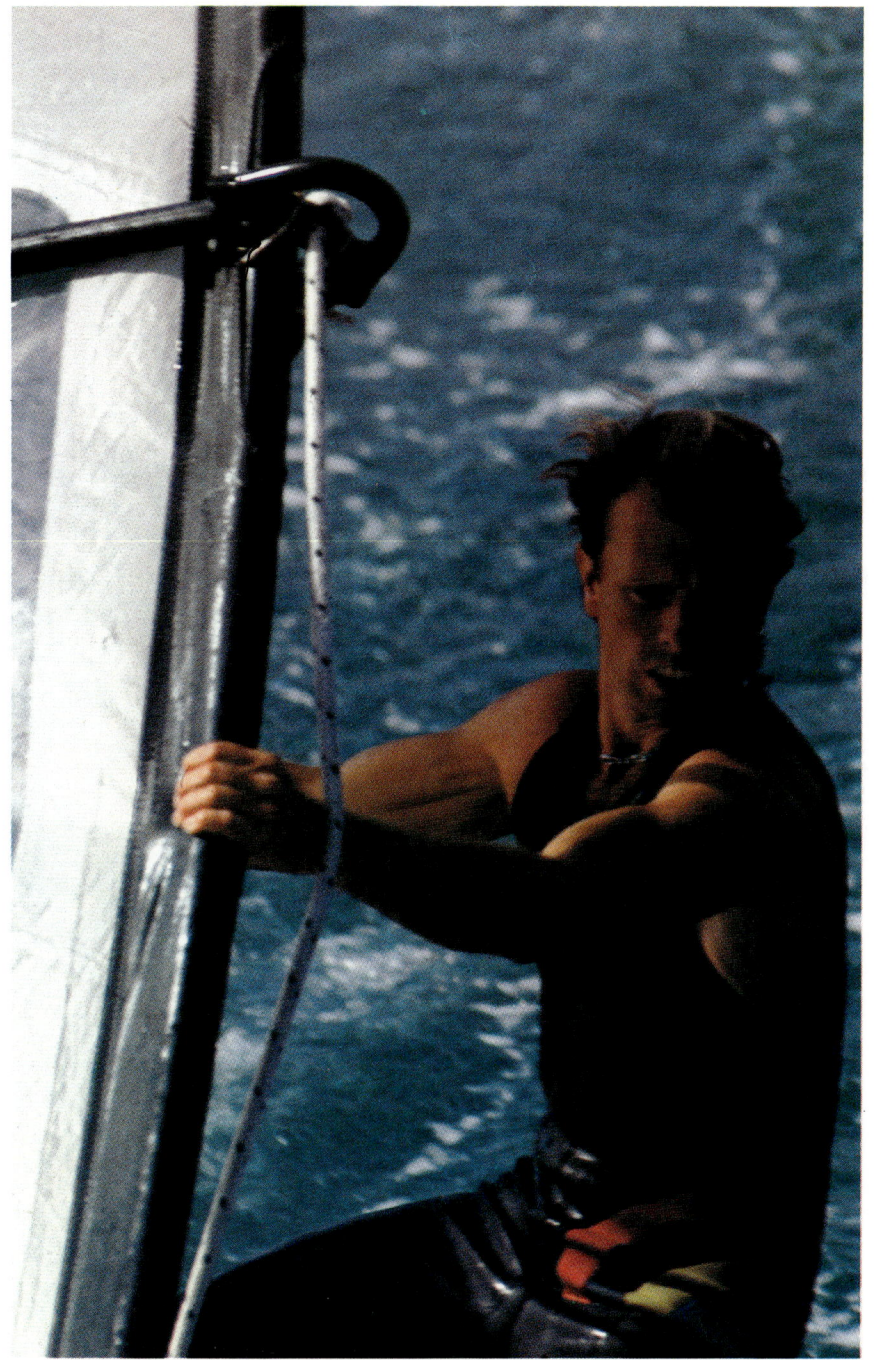

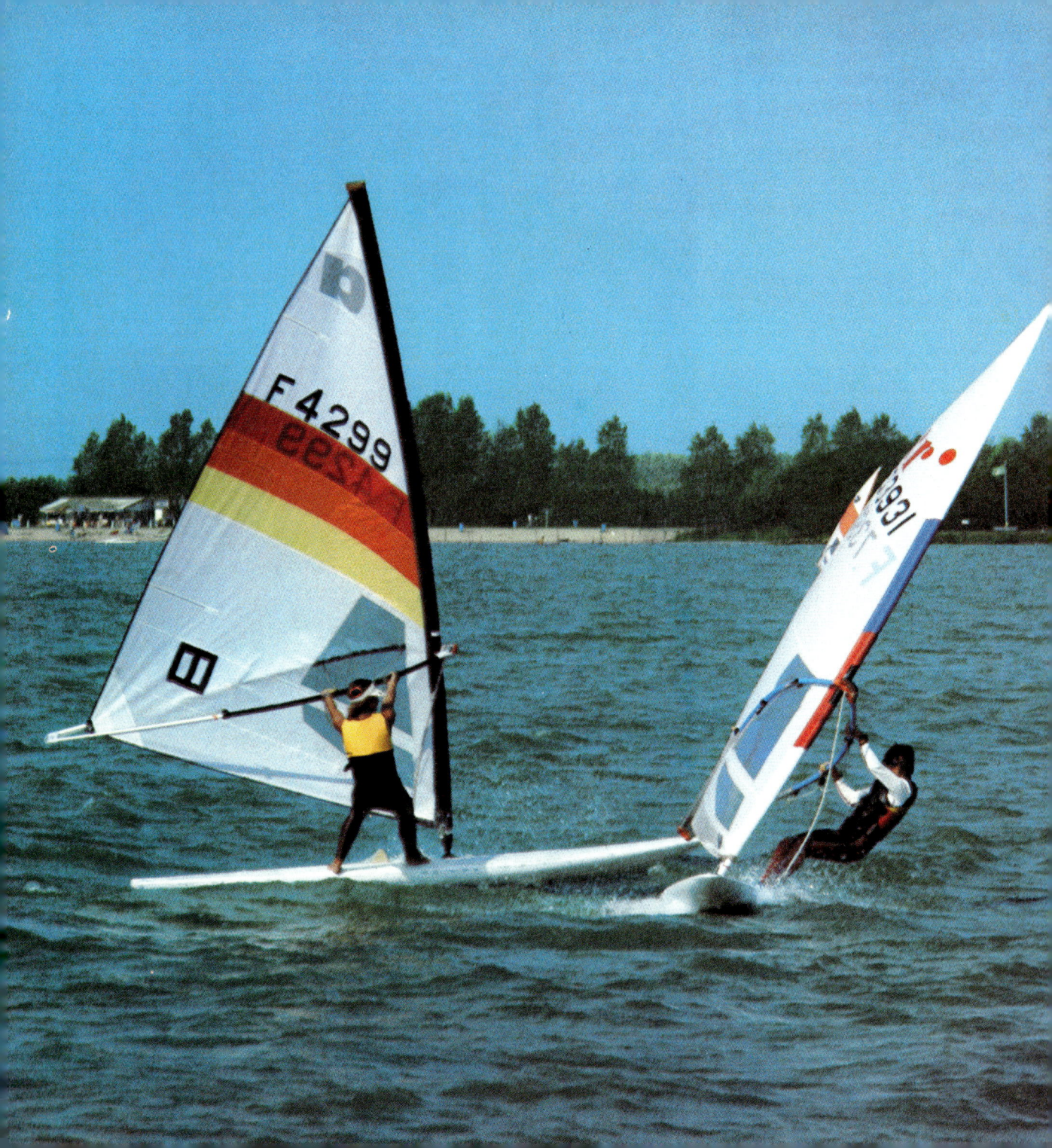

Tacking

If you wish to sail in the direction the wind is coming from, you need to tack. To do this, beat to port and starboard, sailing a zig-zag course to reach the point you wish to get to. The greatest difficulty here is finding the best length for each tack, so we will give you a few tips to help you.

With the wind blowing steadily, make as few turns as possible; each turn costs you speed and time.

When you are facing away from the point you wish to get to, i.e. when it is abeam, it is time to turn, because from now on, you can sail directly towards it.

When the wind speed is low, allow for the leeway force, which would make you drift away.

If the wind alters to blow more from abeam, head up and take advantage of that shift. If it starts to blow more onto your bow and to head you then must bear off, and if it blows from dead ahead it is time to tack before you come to a dead stop. You cannot sail directly into the wind. The nearest you can get is about 45° to the wind direction.

If the point you wish to get to is not directly to windward, one distinguishes between the direct tack and the cross tack. On the direct tack, you sail towards the point you are trying to reach. On the cross tack you get into the best position for sailing towards where you want to be. Always make the direct tack longer than the cross tack.

All in all, tacking requires a great deal of practice.

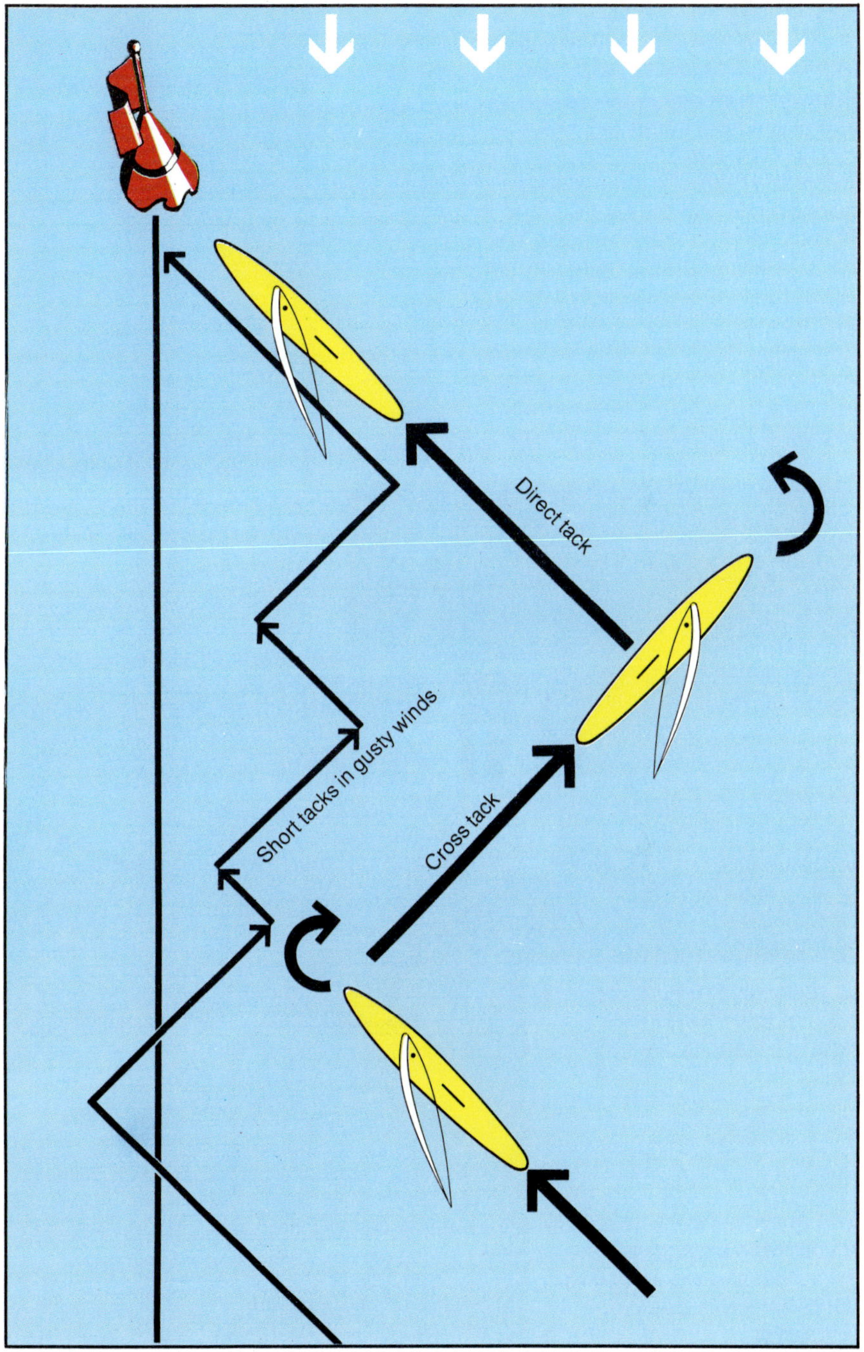

◀ *Two roundboards tacking*

Direct tack

Short tacks in gusty winds

Cross tack

Gybing

For gybing, too, we have two series of photographs to illustrate two different methods. Each sequence runs from right to left.

The "fast gybe" differs from the beginner's gybe in the dynamic support given to the turning motion by putting weight on the edge and stern, and by continuing to turn on the old side of the sail until one is on the new reach. As with the fast turn (see page 32ff), the slow, unsteady method of continuing to turn by inclining the sail into the wind is replaced by a different technique.

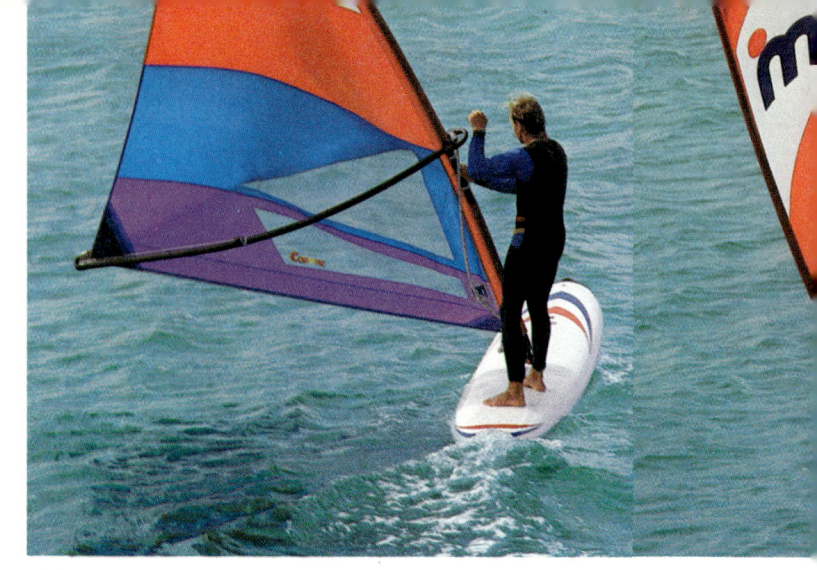

Move sheet hand to mast and immediately pull rig well to windward

Continue turning until on new reach. Pull rig to windward and move off ▲

The board turns more quickly if you keep your arm stretched and the clew only just above the surface of the water ▶

36

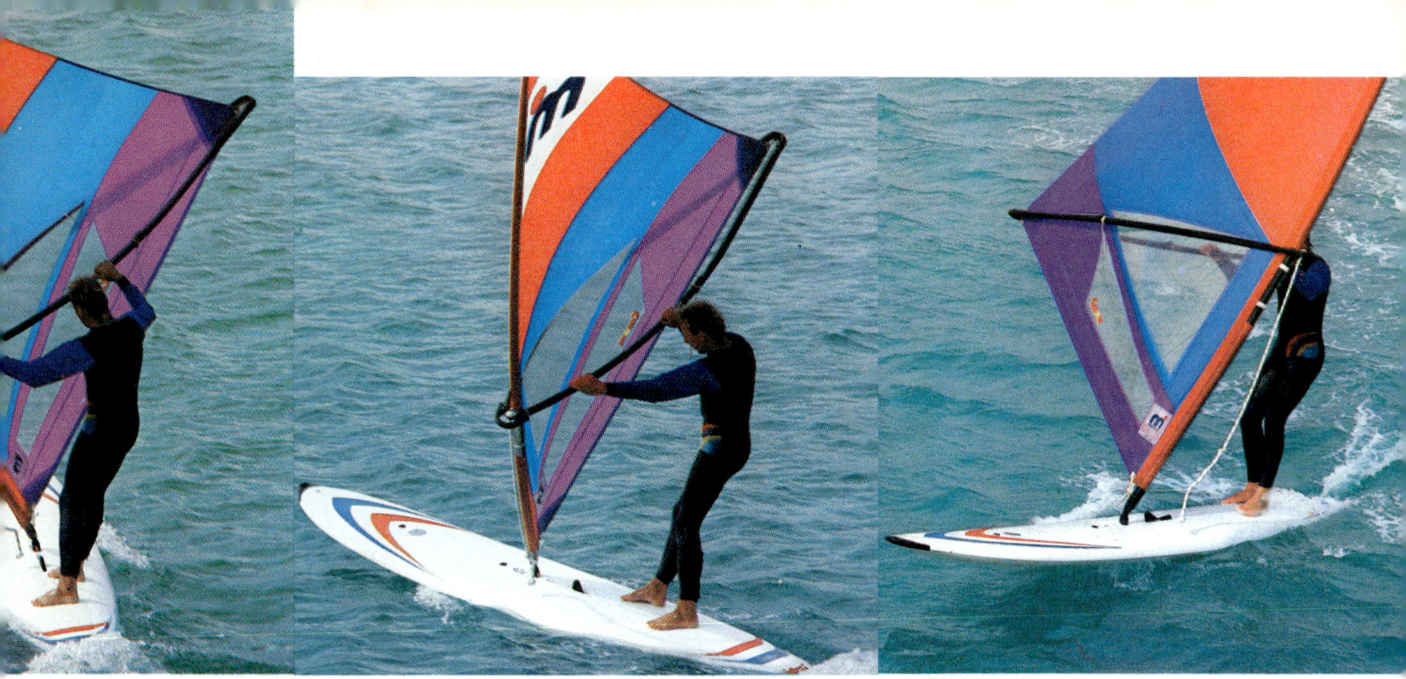

Continue turning keeping clew forward and putting weight on outer edge

Move sheet hand to mast, let sail swing round

Continue turning until stern has passed through eye of wind, and change position of feet

When board is running, change position of feet

To bear away quickly, put weight on outer edge and stern

Bear away by inclining rig to windward and tilting it towards the water

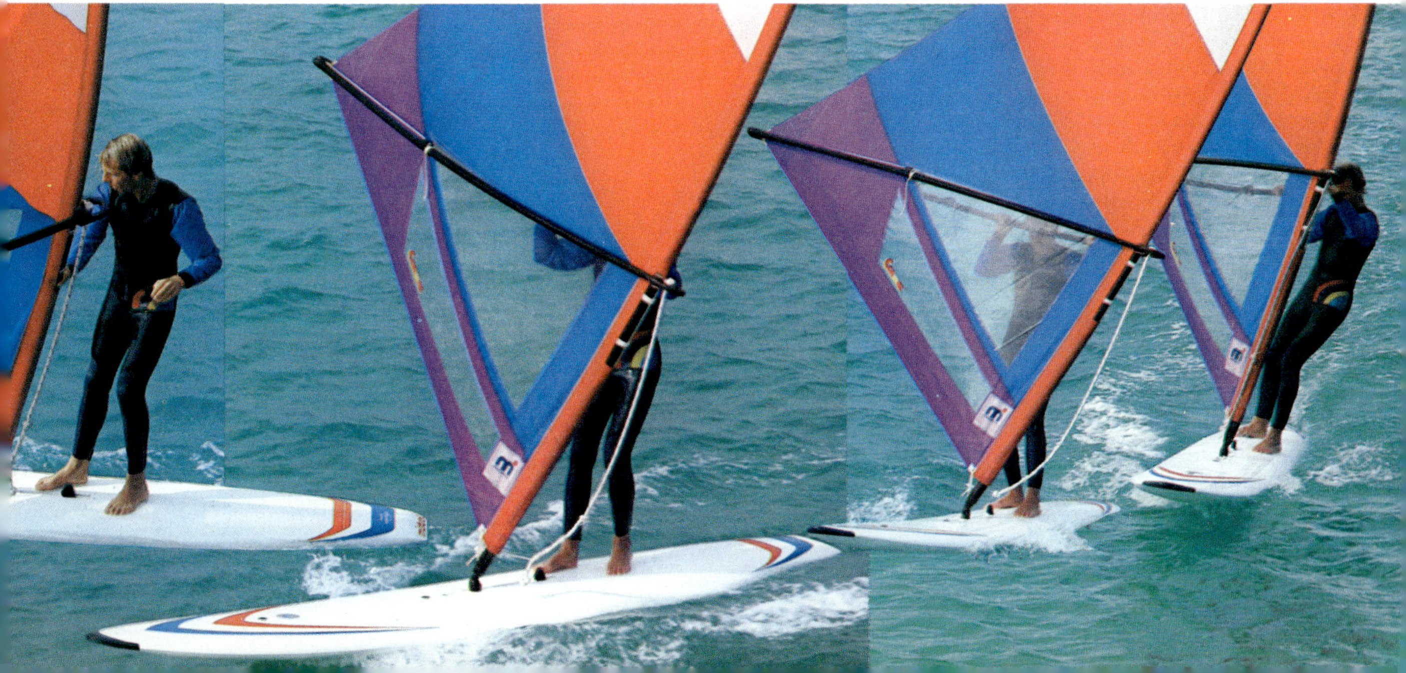

The various stages of the beginner's gybe

- Bear away until running.
- Move back foot forward and front foot back.
- Take hold of mast with sheet hand.
- Continue turning the board by inclining the sail into the wind.
- Lower the clew considerably.
- Turn until initial position is reached.
- Move off.

For the fast gybe, you must

- support the turning motion by putting weight on the outer edge and stern (even in a strong wind, you will not lose much headway)
- continue turning with clew pointing forward until on the new reach
- move sheet hand to mast and pull rig hard, well over to windward
- move off again at once with mast hand on mast.

When you have mastered the beginner's gybe and want to learn the fast gybe as a useful and at the same time exciting manoeuvre, we would recommend you to carry out the exercises on this and the opposite page frequently.

These exercises also fulfil another purpose, though: when you have to take avoiding action, you will often find yourself compelled to swing to windward to do so, i.e. to head up. You will prefer to do that, anyway, as you will no doubt have discovered that bearing away quickly involves a number of problems. However, if you can bear away quickly, within a matter of yards with practice, you will find that you will enjoy the movement and the feeling of being in control of your board, and at the same time you will be much safer.

Exercises

- Sail on a run. If you step well back from the daggerboard case, you will be able to steer your board by putting your weight on one of the edges (see illustrations 2 and 3). The further back you go, the more sensitively your board will react to the weight on the edge. When the wind is fairly strong, keep your arms bent; if the wind drops, stretch your arms again (illustration 1).
- Sail on a reach. If you now alternately put your weight first on one edge of your board and then

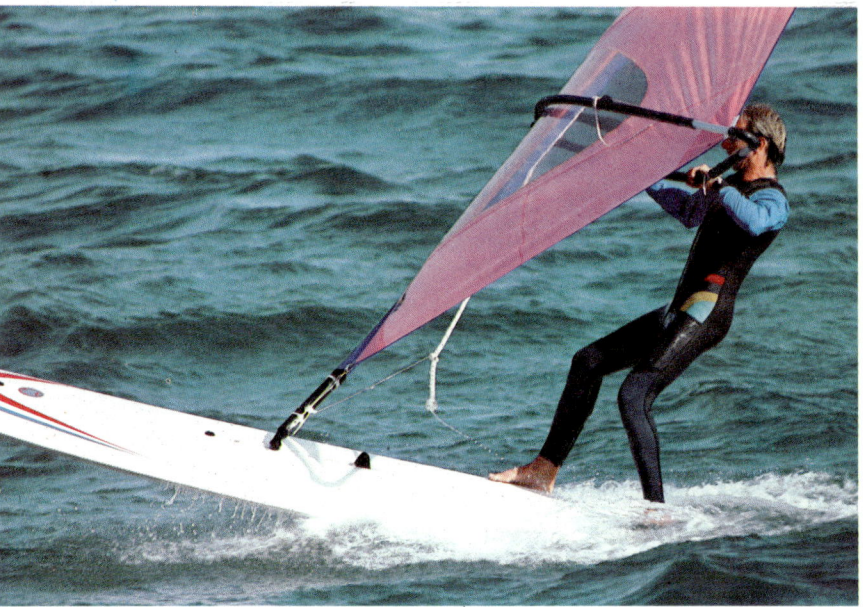

▲ 1   ▼ 2   ▼ 3

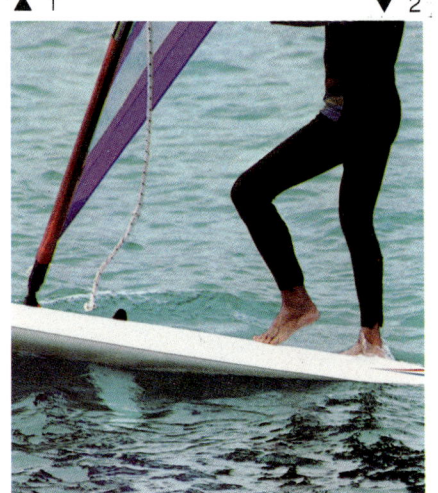
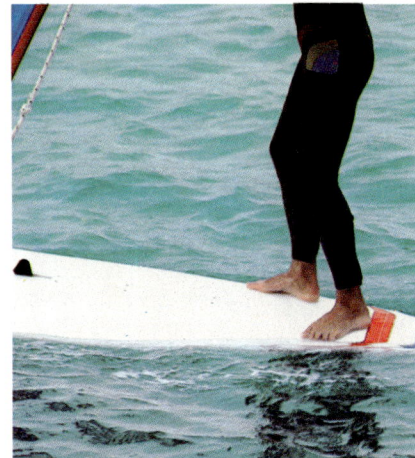

on the other, it will turn gently. During this exercise, make sure that your sail remains in exactly the same position while you try tilting the board, otherwise two ways of steering will coincide: either rig and edge-steering will combine to increase each other's effect, or they will cancel each other out (illustration 5).

● Sail on a reach. Tilt your rig slightly to leeward (clew down) and at the same time put your weight on the windward edge. Two methods of steering are now in opposition to each other:
   ○ the rig steering (to leeward) forces the board to head up
   ○ the edge-steering (putting weight on the windward edge) forces the board to bear away.
The two methods will cancel each other out if they are equally strong.

● Sail on a reach. Leave the rig where it is, and move your feet as far back as you can towards the stern, until you can only just keep the board on a reach (illustration 4).

● Steering with the rig, sail in a wavy line, and remain behind the daggerboard case all the time.

● Increase these wavy lines by putting your weight on the appropriate edge:
   ○ to bear away: put your weight on the windward edge,
   ○ to head up: put your weight on the leeward edge.

● Bear away until running. Continue turning until you are sailing with the clew forward. Try to sail some distance like this, and only then let the sail swing round (illustration 6).

● In as short a space as possible, perform as many gybes as you can, one after the other.

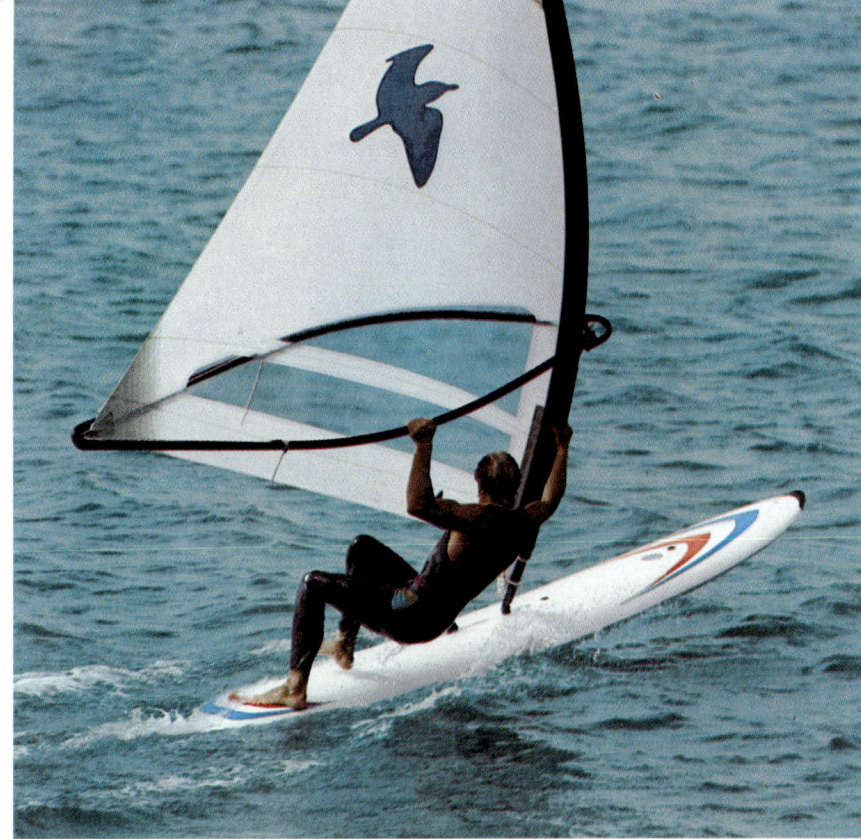

▲ 4

▼ 5

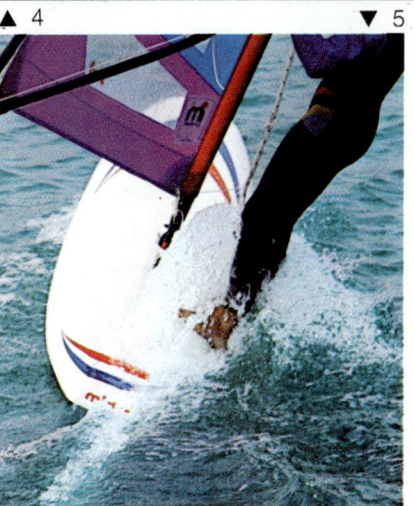

▼ 6

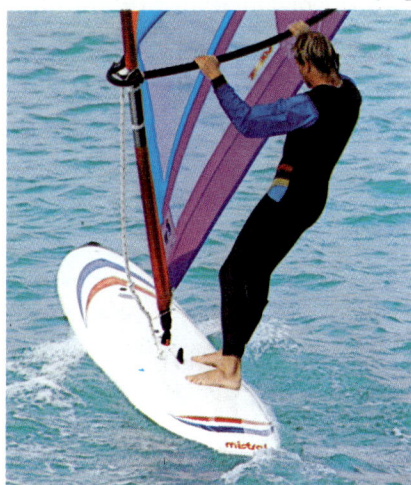

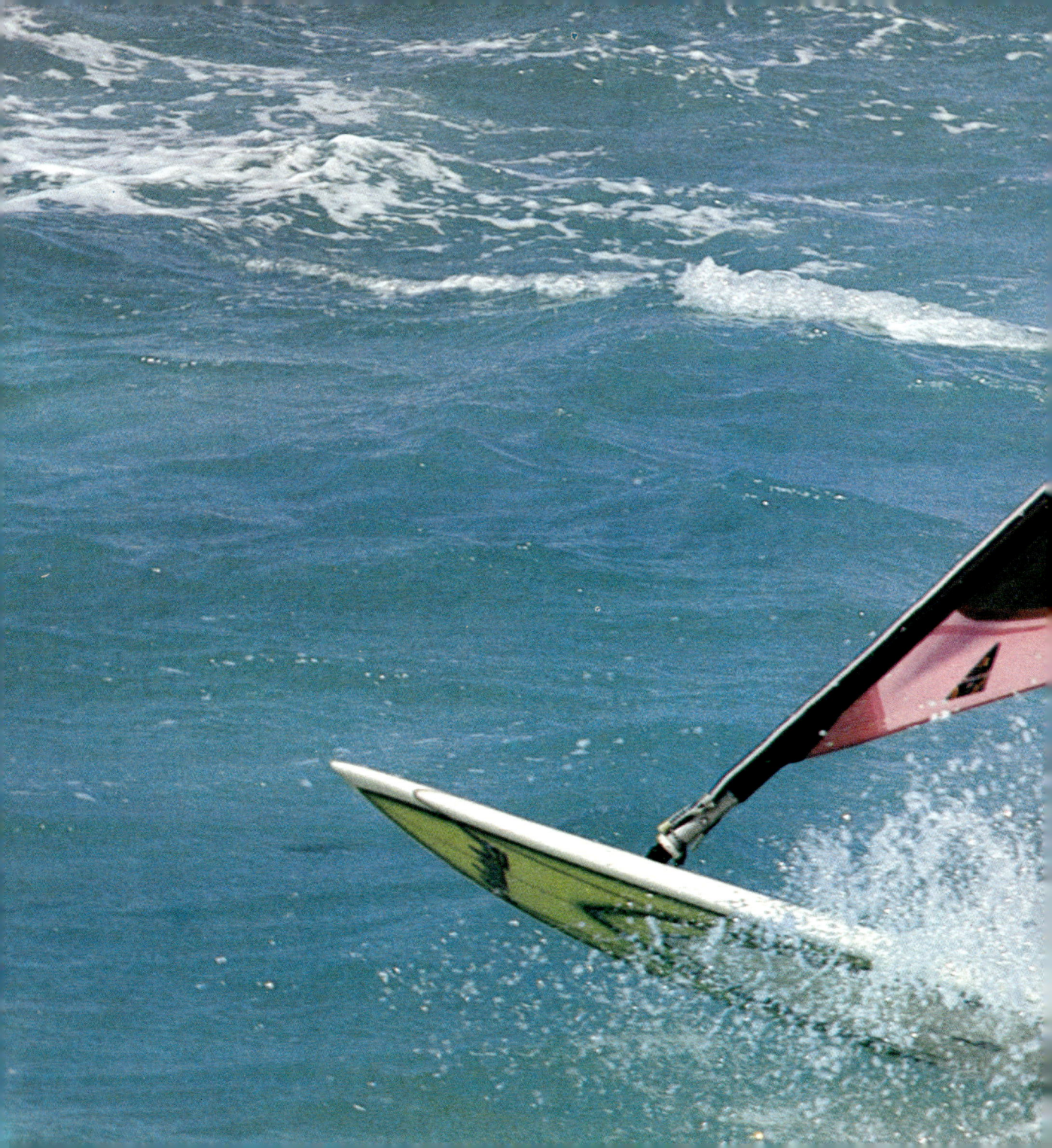

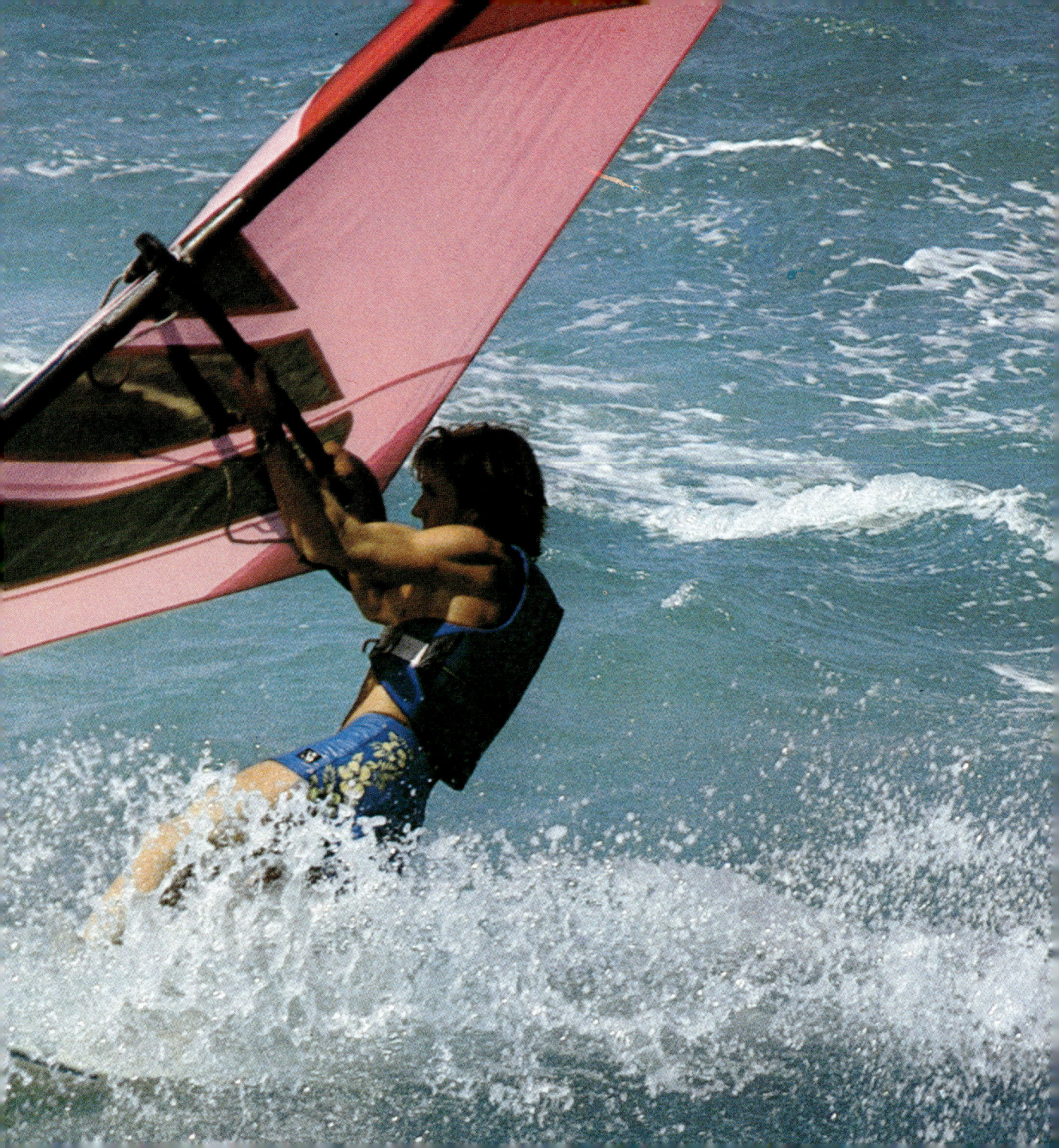

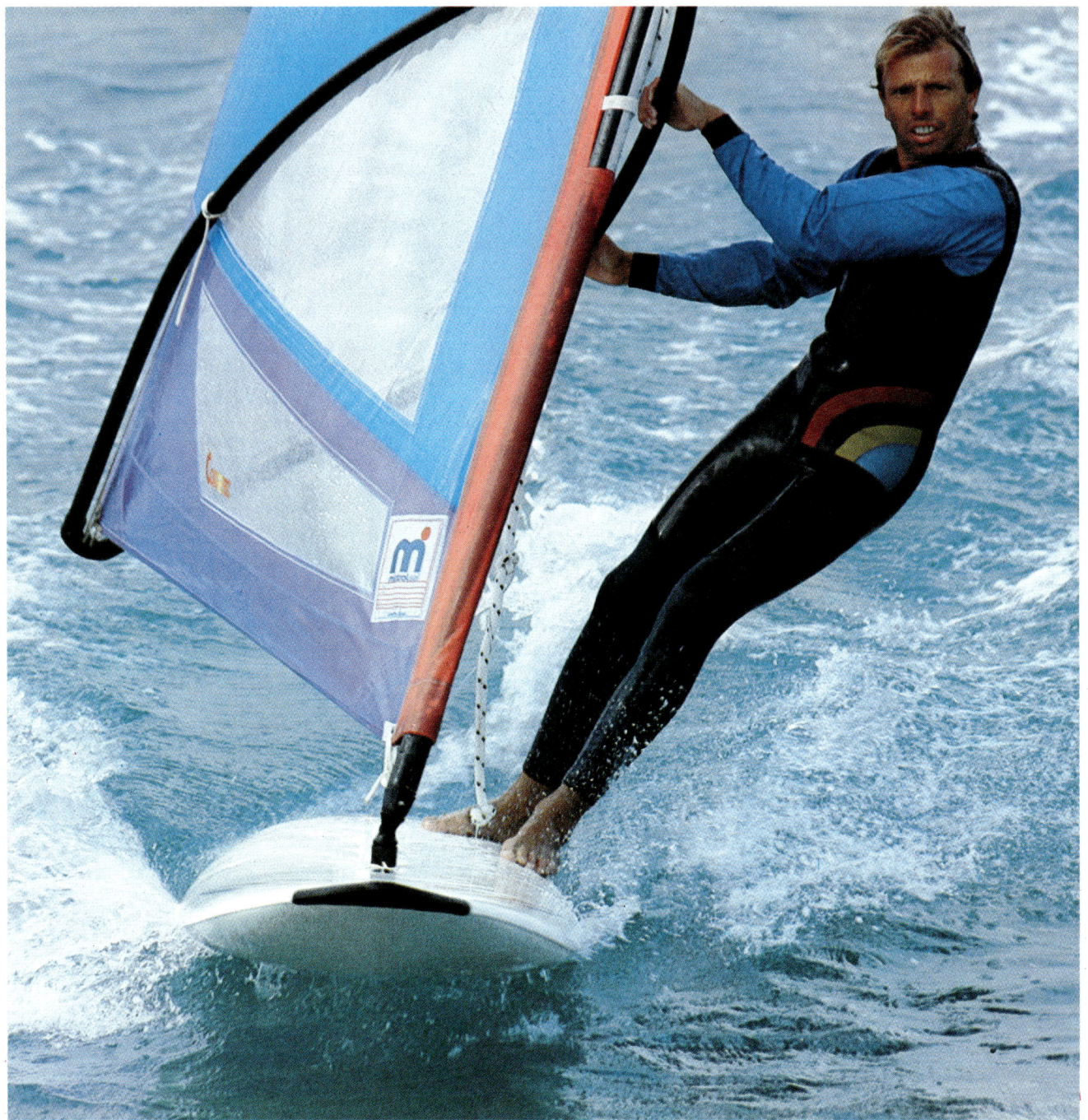

Windsurfing with a minimum of effort

Many people think of windsurfing as a heavy form of exercise. Naturally, there would be no point in telling you that it takes no physical effort at all. But if you get your technique right, the effort will be far less than you might think. Good technique involves primarily the proper sail position (with the arm and body relaxed) as well as optimum board and sail trim.

Most effort is wasted by using the wrong sail position. If you want to find out the best sail position, you should have a look at the different positions of a sail in relation to the wind: when you take hold of the rig near the mast and let it blow freely, it will head to the wind and flap. If you then sheet in a little bit, it will start to fill up, beginning at the leech. The more you sheet in, the closer to the mast the sail will flap. When it has just disappeared at the mast, then your sail has reached the correct position.

If you continue to sheet in at this point, it will feel as though the sail drive is increasing. It is in fact decreasing, but acting at right angles to the board instead of propelling it. If you have a look at the illustrations you will understand what this means.

If you have got your sail in the correct position and still want to save energy, you should hang your weight to windward as soon as the wind permits. Then — and not before — you can stretch out your arms.

If you now let the rig hang to leeward, you will head up naturally.

Your hands should be placed on the wishbone, a shoulder-width apart and at equal distances from the Centre of Effort, so that you can counteract any veering of the wind

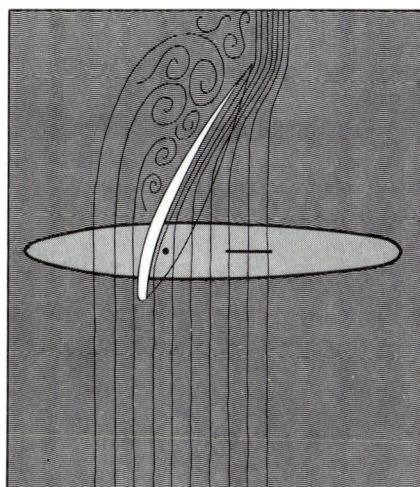

Oversheeting: the air flow becomes turbulent

without any arm effort, merely by turning round. The tension should be equal on both arms. Try surfing

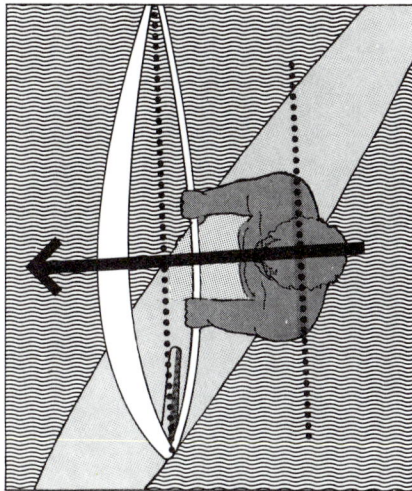

Forces act on body symmetrically

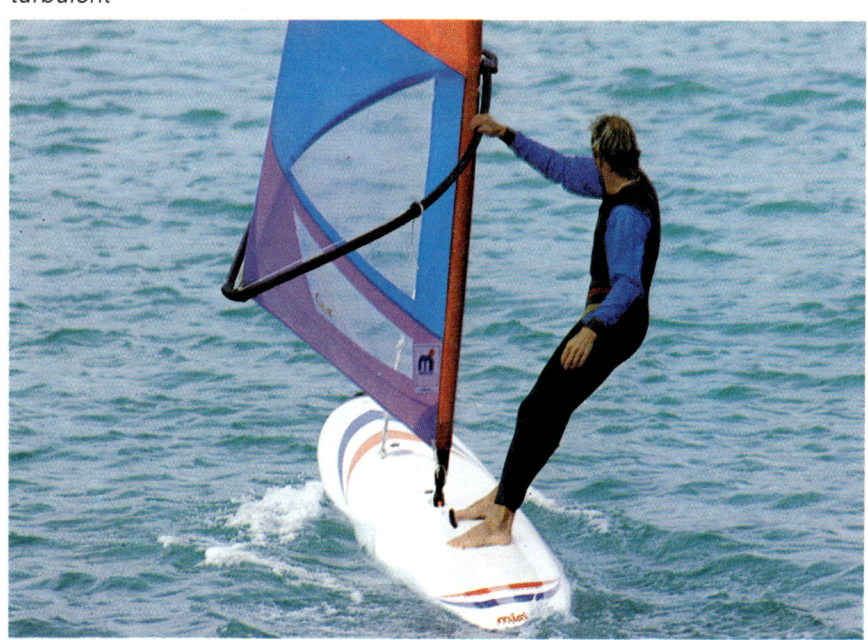

Surfing with one hand. Gradually move your hands together on the wishbone until you can feel the Centre of Effort. Then let go with one hand.

with one hand. In moderate winds this is not too difficult.

Correct *body posture* is another way of saving energy: of course, you need to keep your body flexed at all times if you want to avoid losing control of your body's centre of gravity. But if you stretch your body, without moving your hips, this basic position will hardly require any effort and you can always use your weight to balance the effect of the wind.

Keep your feet as wide apart as your hips, placing the tips of your toes at right angles to the sail.

In this way your board will move fast without requiring much effort.

Exercises

● Travelling on one leg
● Travelling with legs straddled
● Travelling in a half-kneeling position

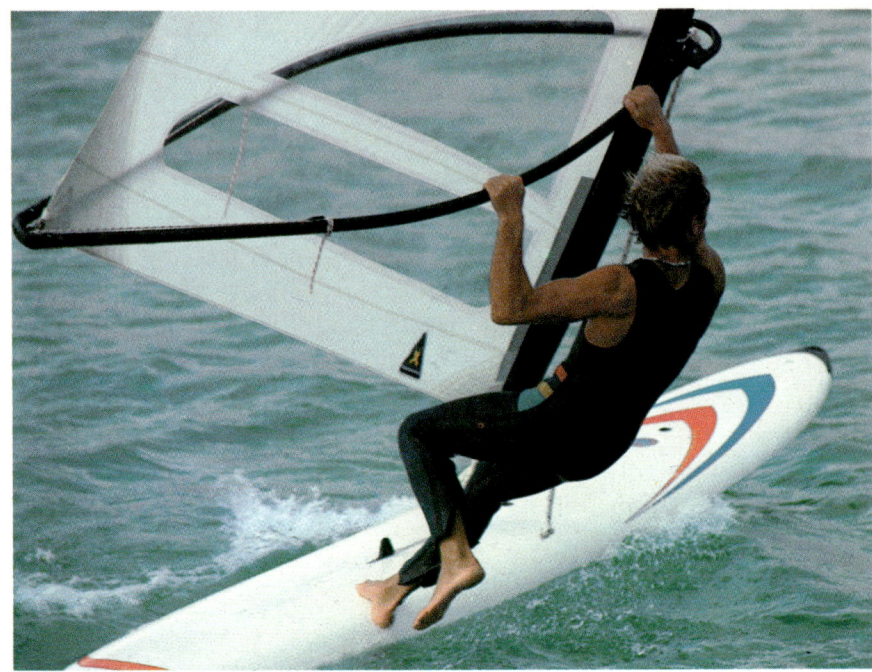

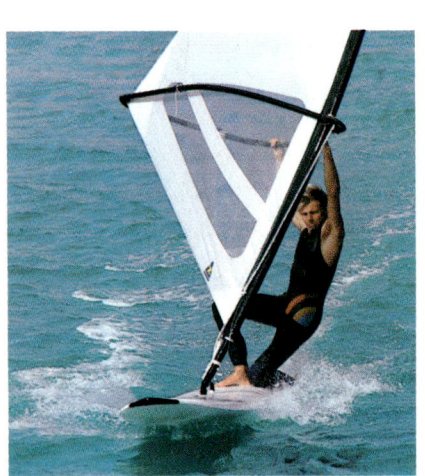

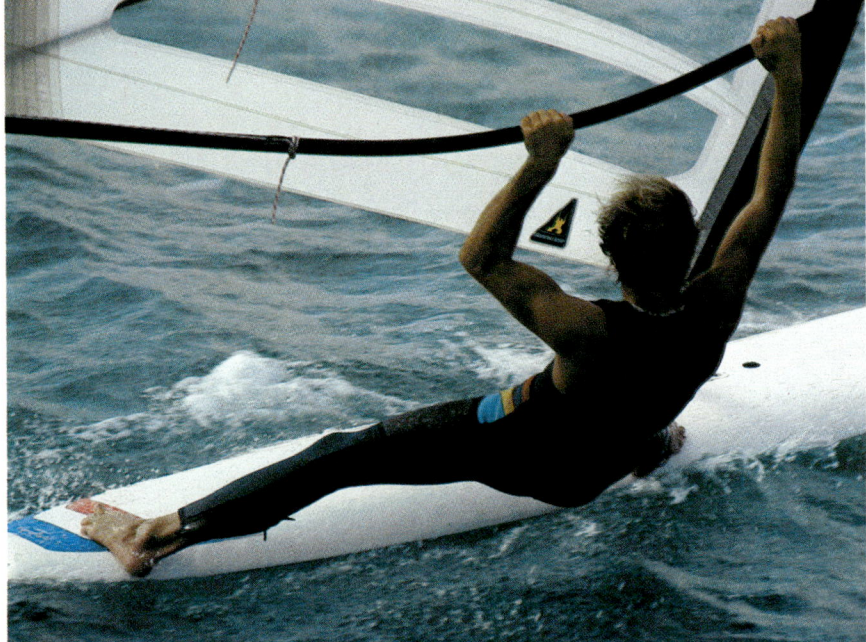

The beach start

In the chapter on "Carrying the board to the water" (page 16), we showed you how to carry your board to the water without causing any damage to your equipment or inconveniencing people in the water.

The same goes for the beach start, a technique which is somewhat more elegant and seamanlike. Even for a beach start you carry your board to the water-line. Depending on your own individual skills, the layout of the shore and the type of waves, you should either put your board and rig together in the water or choose the "classic" method of introducing them one after another. In the following situations you should put your board and rig in the water separately:
- rocky shores
- when the sea bed drops away sharply
- if other surfers or bathers might be disturbed by a beach start.

In all other situations you can beach start. The most suitable situation is a gently sloping sand beach with few or no waves on the shore and no direct onshore or offshore breezes. When the wind is blowing directly onshore, or when there are two-foot waves breaking directly on the shore, a beach start will be very difficult.

Beach start technique

With an ideal slanting onshore wind, you should carry out the following procedure:
- Place the board at the water-line and insert the mast foot. For safety reasons the sail should be in a leeward position. Do not forget your safety line.
- Take hold of the mast just above the wishbone and move to the windward side of the board, while holding the rig in your hand and the mast in front of you.
- Take hold of the mast with your mast hand and the stern with the hand which is to be your sheet hand. Lift the board, and you are in the initial position.
- Now slide the board into the water. Make sure that your board cuts the waves exactly. You can steer the board if you either push the bow to leeward or pull it to windward with your mast hand — or even more easily if you take a step to the left or right while holding the skeg in your hand (see picture below).
- Watch the approaching waves and bear in mind that the depth of water at the shore may vary considerably.
- When water reaches your knees let the skeg go and grab the wishbone with your sheet hand.
- Put your mast hand on the wishbone too, and push the bow out of the wind until your board is reaching.

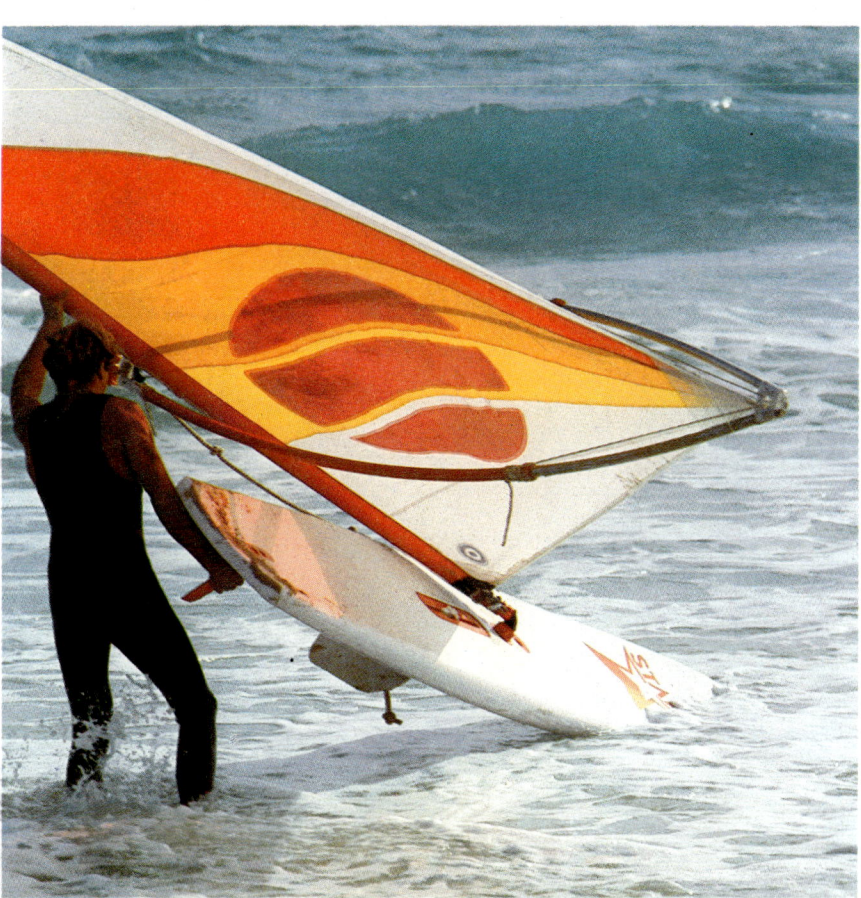

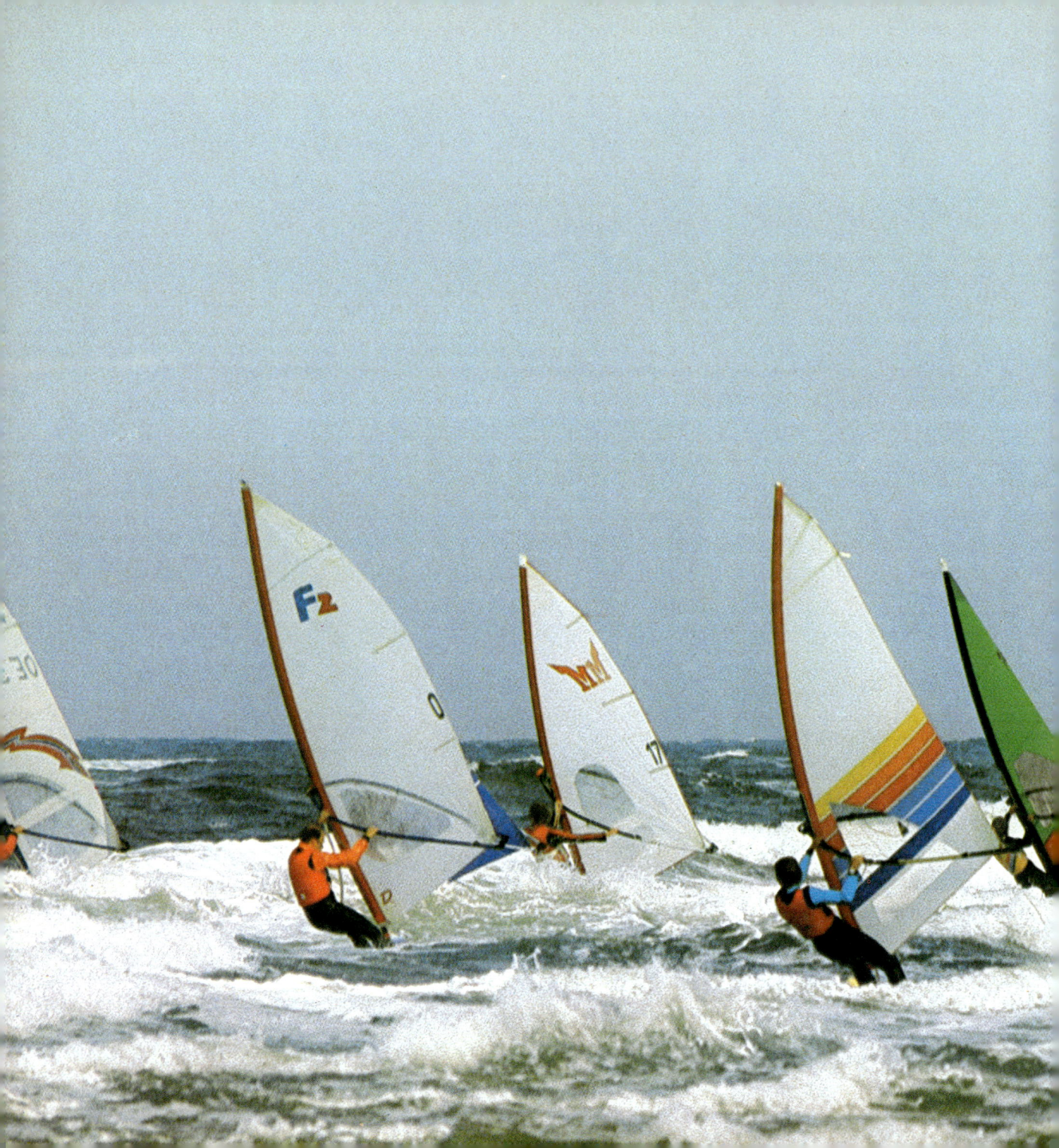

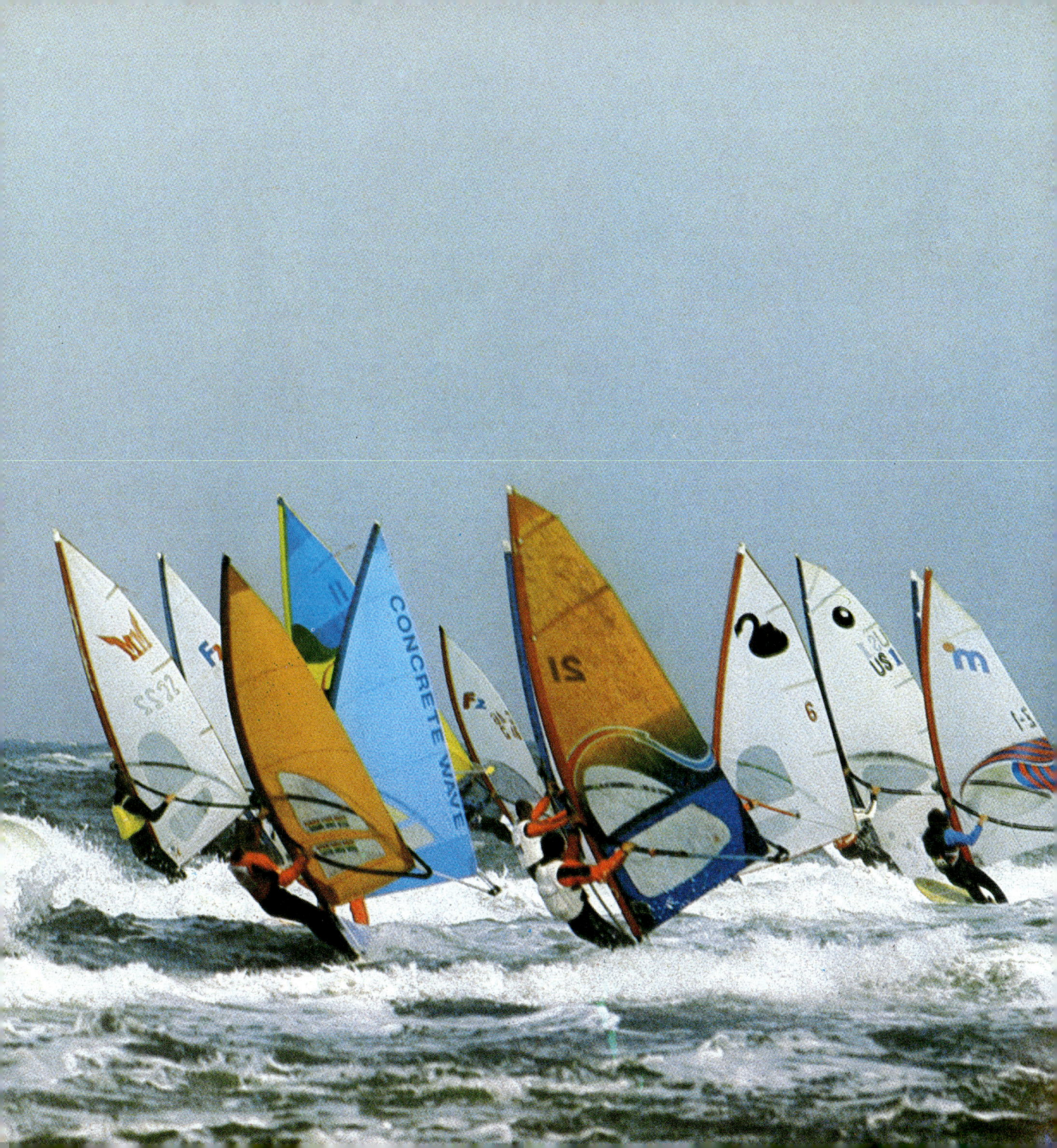

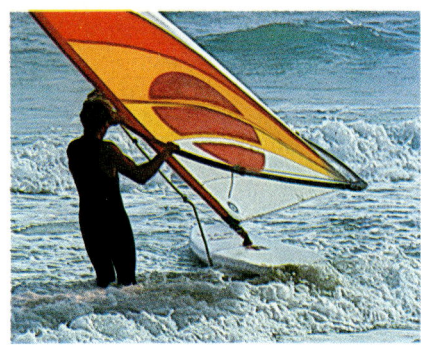

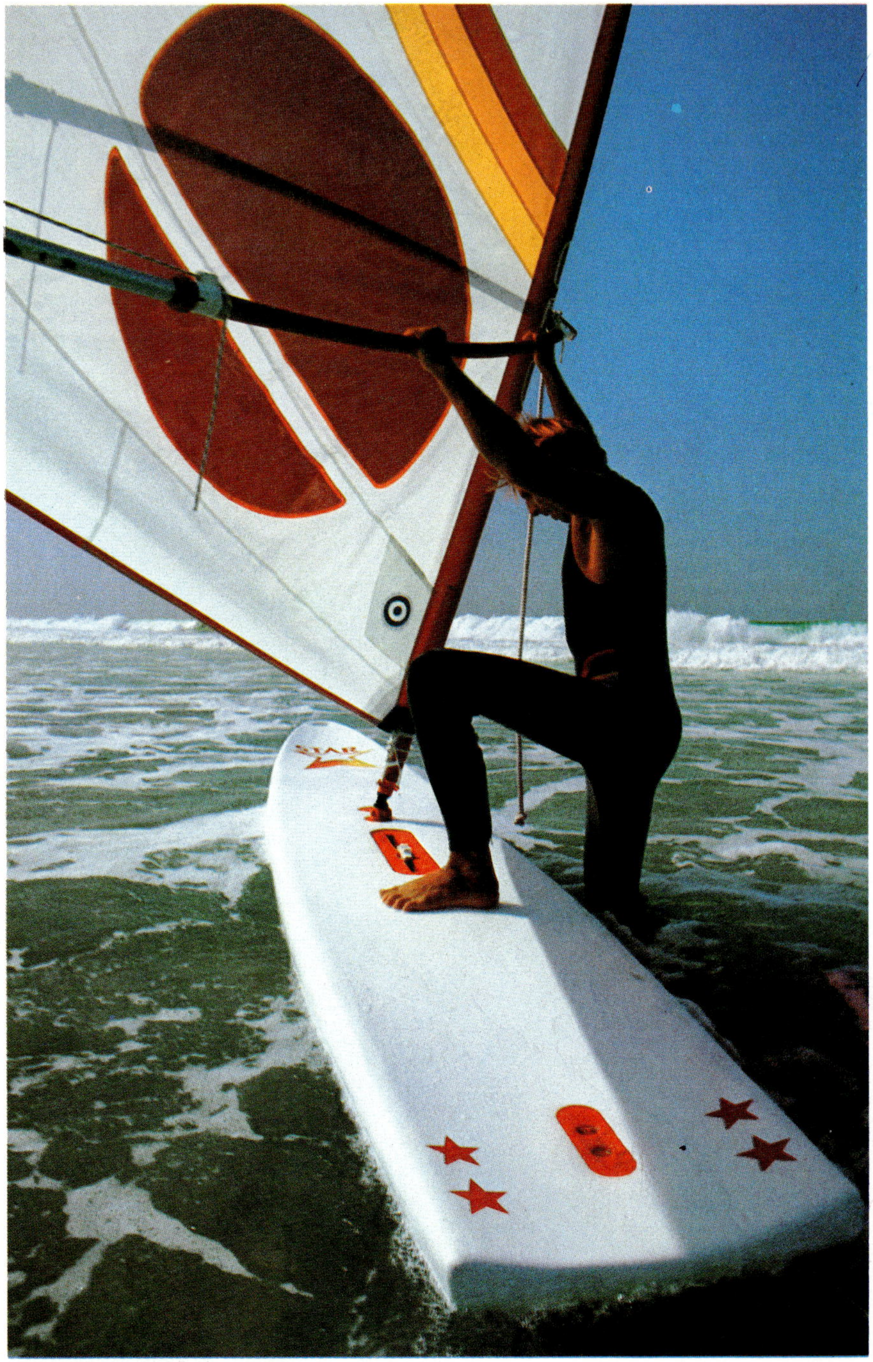

● Step on to the board with your back leg first, and try immediately to get your weight directly above the board. At the same time, sheet in and start sailing. If you take care to keep the wishbone in a horizontal position as you step on, your start will have been successful.

You will find the beach start quite easy in the appropriate situation, but often the circumstances do not allow it. You should therefore practise the start in calm water as often as you can, even when the wind is only light.

Exercise

Stand in calm water on the windward side of your board and

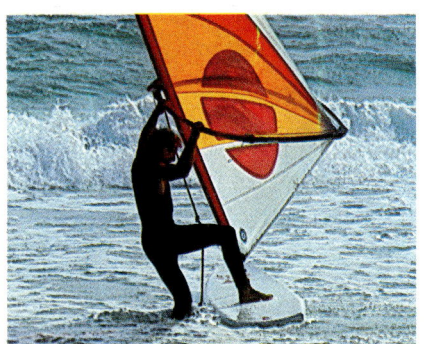

hold the sail with your hands on the wishbone. Even in this position, you can steer your board by leaning the rig sideways. If you lower the clew towards the water it will head up, and if you move forward at an angle towards the mastfoot while lifting the clew it will bear away. The best possible sail position is essential here. Remember to sheet in only to the point where the sail has not yet started to flap.

We suggest that you stay near to the rear third of your board. If you move too far forward, the wind may snatch the sail out of your hand.

Landing

For the sake of any bathers who might be swimming near the beach, for your own convenience and for the protection of your equipment, you should approach the beach *slowly*. Luff up before you reach the point where you intend to get down from the board; otherwise you will end up making a quick landing on the beach, which is hilarious but not very dignified.

Just before you reach the beach, step down backwards and to windward at a point where you expect the sea to be shallow. Leave your masthand on the wishbone. Just as with starting, grab the skeg with your sheethand and push the whole unit on to the beach. If you want to be perfect, just turn the board until the bow is pointing towards the water, deposit the sail on the leeward side and release the downhaul and outhaul lines. This helps to protect both board and sail and prevents the rig from flying in the air. Everything will now be lying ready and waiting for you to make another trip.

Safety in windsurfing

Windsurfers get into severe trouble every year on seas and lakes, and for three main reasons:

- unsuitable or damaged equipment
- overestimation of their own ability
- lack of familiarity with the area.

A windsurfer needs water and wind to enjoy his sport. But as soon as we misinterpret these natural forces, they become a threat to us. Remember at all times that while you can use them to your advantage, you can never impose your will on them; in certain situations they are stronger than man.

You should consult the "Ten Safety Rules" to check what you must always bear in mind if you are to avoid being exposed to avoidable dangers. If you disregard even one of these rules, severe problems may arise. Of course, this does not apply to all kinds of waters. You can go windsurfing alone, and in summer you can even do without your neoprene suit at times if you go to your local gravel pit. However, you should not try to do the same on the open sea. On the exposed North Sea coast, for instance, your first bad experience may also be your last. But let us proceed one step at a time:

1. Get to know the area

Ask other surfers and yachtsmen, or the local surfing school and lifeguards, if any particular dangers are to be expected in the area. In particular, you should be interested in any sudden changes of wind, or of river or tidal currents, reefs and other shallows. Make sure that surfing is permitted on the beach you want to use, and watch out for any driftwood which may rip off your fins.

Ten Safety Rules

1. Find out about the local conditions and regulations.
2. Wear the appropriate warm wetsuit.
3. Check your equipment before every run.
4. Connect the board and rig by means of a safety line and take a towing line with you.
5. Take the time to make a proper assessment of wind and weather. Stay ashore if there is a strong offshore wind.
6. Never go out on a large lake or on the sea without letting other people know.
7. Do not overestimate your own strength. Choose the sail size carefully and take plenty of breaks. Do not carry on surfing until you are completely exhausted.
8. Stay away from waters with heavy commercial shipping.
9. Improve your technique and familiarize yourself with emergency procedures.
10. Stay with your board in any emergency.

2. Wear warm wetsuits

Put the suit on even when the sun is warm and your feet feel the hot sand. A mishap can easily keep you in the water longer than you intend. Even if you are a surfer who rarely or never falls into the water, you will still get wet. The wind will cause your wet skin to get cold due to evaporation, which can cool you down without your even noticing it. Even if you warm up in warm sand every now and then, your main body temperature will still drop, which may be dangerous.

3. Check your equipment

You should do this at all times and in all places. For this reason we have included a relevant checklist in the chapter on "Assembling the Rig" (page 12). The larger the area of water and the less familiar you are with it, the more accurate this check-up should be.

4. Take a safety line and a towing line with you

The safety line connects the board and rig so that they are never accidentally separated. This line should be at least ¼in. thick, elastic, and fastened firmly. If your rig safety line is insufficient it should be replaced. If you occasionally go to, or are planning to go to, areas with breakers, the line should be fixed to some point of the bow so that when the rig is separated, the board turns and points at the breaking wave. The towing line must be at least 20 feet long. You can tie it around the end of the wishbone or the mast, or put it in your back pack. It can be used as a spare line as well.

5. Assess the wind and weather

The best windsurfers always spend fifteen minutes before they start, just watching the wind, waves and weather, even in areas familiar to them. You should bear in mind that it is often difficult to assess the wind speed while you are ashore. You will find this much easier if there are other sailors or surfers on the water.

Choose a free and open location, even if you have to walk a short distance. Hills, dunes, houses or trees tend to deflect the wind or slow it down. With offshore winds, for example, the lee would extend to a distance fifteen to twenty times as long as the obstacle is high. So, if a dune on the beach is sixty feet high, the normal offshore wind will only begin to be felt at a distance of 300 to 400 yards from the shore. With onshore winds, you can only feel the real wind speed at a distance of 160 yards from the shore. This windward barrier effect is very tricky in waters with big waves. If ever you have ever been pushed by incoming waves on to a rocky shore with no wind in your sail, you will know to keep away from wind obstacles, even with onshore winds.

Never rely exclusively on your personal knowledge of the weather. You should always try to catch the latest weather report on the radio or in a newspaper before you set off on the water.

If you notice a thunderstorm coming up or a cold front approaching, follow the advice given in the chapter on weather (pages 93–98). In neither case can you be safely sure of how the wind will develop. So you should always leave the water.

Towing line tied to the end of the wishbone

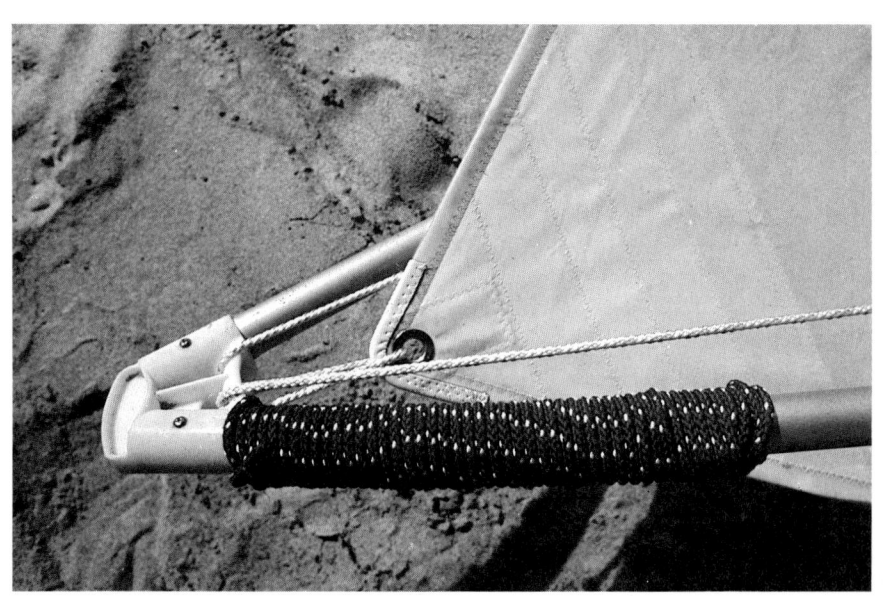

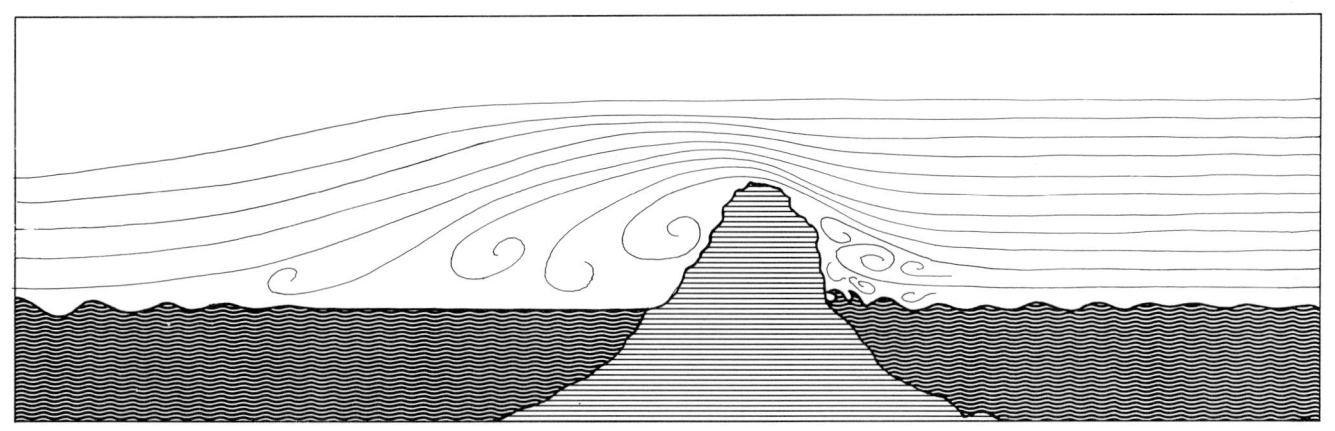

6. Do not sail alone

It is safer and more enjoyable to have someone with you who could help you in an emergency. If you still want to sail on your own on a large lake or on the sea, tell someone on the beach. You should point out the colour of your sail, and tell them the point you are aiming for and the time you intend to come back. In this way, you may be sure that someone will watch you and that help will be available in an emergency.

7. Do not overestimate your abilities

Even if you have taken careful note of the wind and weather conditions, you cannot always be sure of being able to handle them. When in doubt, you should always choose the smaller sail and consider the possibility of refraining from sailing altogether. Such decisions will depend on a variety of different factors. Take your time in considering them. Even if you are sure you can go surfing without any problems, you should go on a short exploratory trip and then return ashore for a break.

8. Stay away from commercial shipping

Commercial shipping vessels will not make way for you, as their size prevents this. Large ships deflect the wind strongly to leeward or windward in the same way as obstacles ashore, and this could cause you to lose your manoeuvrability. If you have had an accident and are drifting in the water, a ship may notice you too late. In such "encounters" the surfer will always come off worst. So you should as a matter of course stay away from all areas where there is likely to be any commercial shipping.

9. Improve your windsurfing technique and be ready to help both yourself and others

The better you can control your board and cope with the physical forces involved in the sport, the smaller will be the risk of your getting into trouble. However, you should know how to help yourself and others in an emergency. Get your friends to practise the salvage

Leeward shelter and the windward barrier effect are very tricky

and towing operations with you (these are explained on page 54). Theoretical knowledge is not enough. In the actual situation you will most often be confronted with difficult conditions and even experienced surfers may have trouble when they have to tow.

10. Stay with your board at all times

As the surfboard is unsinkable, it forms an ideal life raft. Whatever your situation, you will always be better off on your board than trying to swim ashore. You do not cool off so quickly, and by paddling you can move faster and use less energy than by swimming. Furthermore, if both your warm wetsuit and your sail are in flashy colours, you will stand a better chance of being seen by someone. Even the most advanced surfer must be warned against using boards with a volume of less than 100 litres! If you go under this limit you are recklessly endangering your life.

Harness surfing

It is not by accident that this introduction to harness surfing immediately follows the chapter on safety. The harness makes surfing more fun for the proficient sailor and offers an additional *safety reserve* in an emergency. It does not, however, serve to enable sailors who are in bad condition or technically unsure to surf in high winds. You do save energy in your arms and shoulders but the harness will not minimize your efforts. If you do not practise saving energy without the harness, simply by holding your sail in the appropriate position and keeping your body in a relaxed posture, you will get used to sailing in the wrong position, with a tense body posture.

Equipment

Use a harness only if it can be hooked and unhooked without your having to take your hands off the wishbone. There should be one or more buckles which release you from the whole harness as soon as you are lying underneath the sail with the harness line twisted around the hook. A small back pack on the harness would be useful for carrying spare ropes and a spare hook. Harness lines should be made of stiff pre-stretched material, and have a diameter of not less than 1/3 inch.

Attachment

Feel the point on the wishbone where you can hold the rig for a short while with one hand. Attach the two ends of the line 8 to 12 inches to either side of this point. Turn the loose end twice round the wishbone and then tie the end in a figure-of-eight knot once around the

line. The remaining end may be secured by another figure-of-eight knot. By slightly pressing your thumb on it while sailing, you can loosen this attachment and shift it sideways. The line should sag so far that you can travel with your arms almost fully stretched out when you take hold of the wishbone with your hands a shoulder-width apart.

Technique

Your technique should ideally remain the same, whether you are with or without a harness. Only the tension on your arms will, for the most part, be transferred to the lines. However, most harness surfers have their sail sheeted in too far, which is wrong. So check your sail position continually. For this purpose you should unhook occasionally while sailing.

To hook in with the hook opening down, pull the wishbone upwards in a circle towards you with a sharp jerk. The line swings up into the hook. This hooking movement can best be practised on dry land.

To unhook, pull the wishbone towards you until the line falls off. Note that in both cases the sail is moved towards your body, and not vice versa!

When you first start harness surfing, the idea of being attached firmly to the wishbone may make you feel somewhat uneasy. So we have included some exercises which you can easily repeat several times in moderate winds. Then you will soon be able to handle the harness safely. Here again, it is vital to position the sail exactly, and to sheet in and out by turning the upper part of your body.

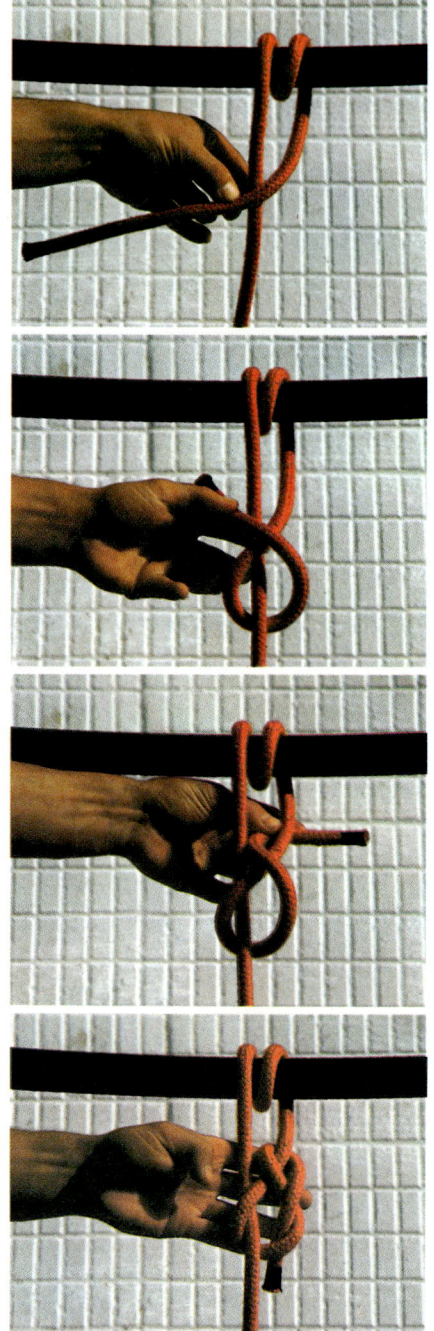

Exercises

● Start sailing without the harness and with your arms slightly bent. Do the stop/go exercise (page 24). Make sure that you sheet in and out *exclusively* by turning your upper body.

● Start sailing with a gentle breeze *inside the wishbone*. That way you can sheet in and out only by turning your upper body.

● When beating, hook in on the harness and allow the sail to pull you into a fall to leeward. If your hands remain on the wishbone, nothing will happen to you.

Repeat this exercise several times, as it will make you feel safer when you fall to leeward.

● Hook in and carefully fall to windward in the harness beneath the sail. Once you are in the water, you simply grab the hook and disengage the line if it has not become unhooked by itself.

● Hook yourself into the harness in a moderate wind, and take first one and then both hands off the wishbone. You will notice that you can sheet in and out with no hands by turning the upper part of your body (see adjacent picture).

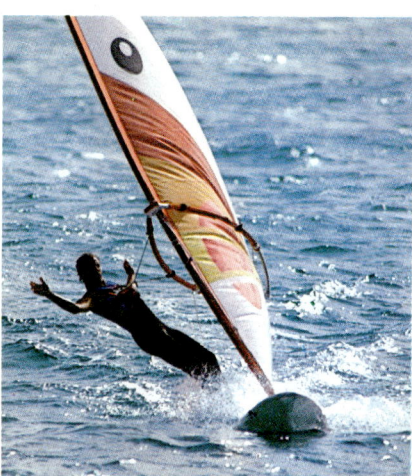

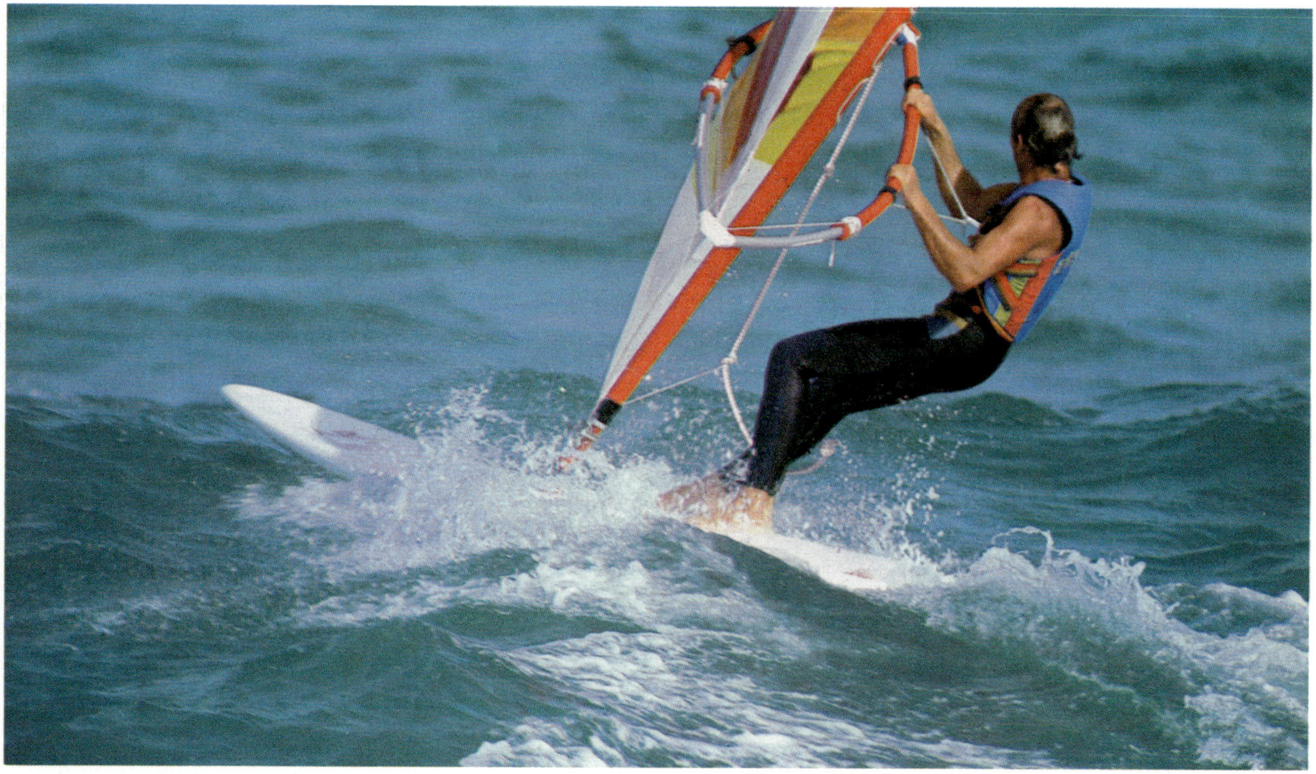

◀ *Attaching the harness line to the wishbone*

Harness surfing means more fun for the proficient surfer

What to do in an emergency

A variety of things may prevent you from sailing back to your starting point. Windless conditions are probably the least problematic, though you cannot manoeuvre in them. The situation can be much more unpleasant if your equipment is damaged, and on top of that you are near exhaustion and the offshore wind is increasing. The solution will depend on the situation. This chapter will tell you what possibilities there are of rescuing yourself and others when in difficulties — what you can do and what you have to know.

You must be familiar with:
● the international distress signals
● methods of provisional repair if equipment is damaged
● towing technique
● the correct procedure for being towed.

If you are in trouble the choice of action you will have to take depends, among other things, on your equipment, the wind speed and direction, the locality, and the techniques you can handle. For example, you should carry a small red (distress) flare and use it if your mast is irreparably broken on the open sea with a strong offshore wind, unless you are in the immediate vicinity of the shore. If you are on a small lake with moderate winds or at sea with direct onshore winds, you need not give the signal. Instead you should either make provisional repairs, wait until you drift ashore or paddle home.

International distress signal without any devices

Besides distress signals included in the international code (such as orange smoke, red distress flares or the flags NC), there is a distress signal which is known around the world and which obliges everybody to help immediately as long as this does not endanger them too. This duty to render assistance is laid down by law. When you are in an emergency, *and only then*, sit or kneel on your board and make the signal calmly and clearly so that it can be correctly interpreted.

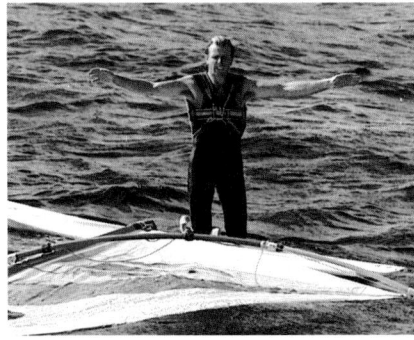

Distress signal: raise and lower your extended arms

Provisional repairs to damaged equipment

In the following cases of seriously damaged equipment, you can help yourself with a provisional repair or with a special technique in not too difficult situations — this is assuming you are unable to pull down the rig and paddle ashore. For any broken harness lines you should always have a spare line with you.

Broken mast. Remove the sail and insert the top of the mast upside down in the lower part. As the mast is now shorter, you can hardly trim the sail, so pull it carefully over the mast. In most cases this will be sufficient to get you ashore.

Broken wishbone. If the wind is not too high you can return with the help of that part of the wishbone which has remained intact. Otherwise you have to pull down the rig and paddle, or maybe launch a distress signal.

Clew torn off. Tie the clew by means of a sheet bend (page 78) to a spare end of the outhaul line. If the clew is very high up on your sail, you will find it difficult to manage this knot. In any case you will end up with a very provisional sail.

Broken fin. If there are several fins on your board, this damage is not very serious. If your board has a daggerboard and one fin only you can still control the board by pushing on the leeward side. If your board has nothing more than one fin you will have to paddle home.

Broken daggerboard. The most common daggerboard fracture occurs on the lower edge of the daggerboard case. Recover the broken part and insert it in the case from above after you have removed the old head piece. It would be advisable to jam the remaining piece of daggerboard in the case with the spare line.

Broken mast foot or mast foot joint. A short line can be used to connect the downhaul line to a stable anchorage point or the rig safety line on the board.

Packing up for salvage

Packing up the rig for salvage is not even easy when ashore. On the water, an experienced sailor will find it really difficult. As you have to take in the rig in almost every emergency, you could well practise it as a game, or in competition with other surfers. You can do this as follows:

- Sit astride the board, release the rig safety line and take the mast foot out of the board.
- Pull the wishbone end towards you and undo the outhaul line on one side. The other side will remain lashed on.
- Push the end of the wishbone well up the mast. Then, starting at the foot, roll the sail up tightly.
- Remove the battens (if any) and wrap the sail around them. Undo the uphaul line and, starting at the wishbone, wrap it tightly around the mast and sail towards the masthead.
- With the free end of the outhaul line, lash the wishbone to the mast and wrap the remaining outhaul line around the mast and sail, in the direction of the mast foot.

If you want to paddle, put the stowed rig on the board and then lie on top of it. This means that there is no part of the rig touching the water, which could otherwise slow you down.

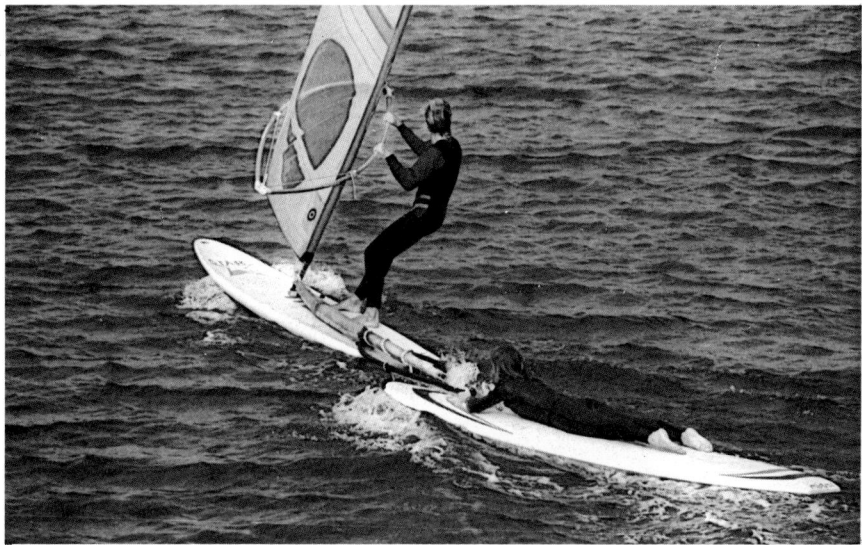

Towing

There are four ways of towing a surfer in distress. Which way you choose will depend on the circumstances and on the equipment.

Towing with a bar

The stowed rig belonging to the surfer in distress is placed in the rear mast foot well of the towing surfer's rig or connected to his downhaul line. The surfer being towed holds tight to his own board and rig.

Towing with a rope

The rope is fixed to the mastfoot of the tower's board and to the tow hook of the board being towed. The longer the rope, which should ideally be about twenty feet long, the greater the safety distance and the fewer problems will arise. The recovered rig is again placed in towing surfer's mast foot well.

Towing by the daggerboard strap or the footstrap

The towed surfer grabs the daggerboard strap or one foot strap of the tower's board. He should be on the windward side of the tower's board so that he will not be injured should the mast come down. This method of towing is only a last resort for when the other methods are impossible due to inappropriate or missing equipment.

Towing with the rig trailing

In very difficult situations such as high waves or winds, or when there is not time for proper stowing of the rig, the surfer in distress simply undoes his outhaul, letting the rig

Towing with a bar

trail behind him. For reasons of safety, towing in such difficult situations should always be carried out with a long enough line.

Have a towing line with you and practise the emergency towing operation in realistic conditions.

Some tips on towing

If you are towing, remember that your sail has to cope with double the weight. So you must go carefully, sheeting in step by step and luffing again when the tension gets too high. Look back several times to ensure that your 'companion' is lying safely on his board. As you are towing a person in distress *all other small vessels* have to give way.

When you are being towed, concentrate on clinging to your board. You may remove your daggerboard so that your board does not work independently and keeps exactly to the towing surfer's path.

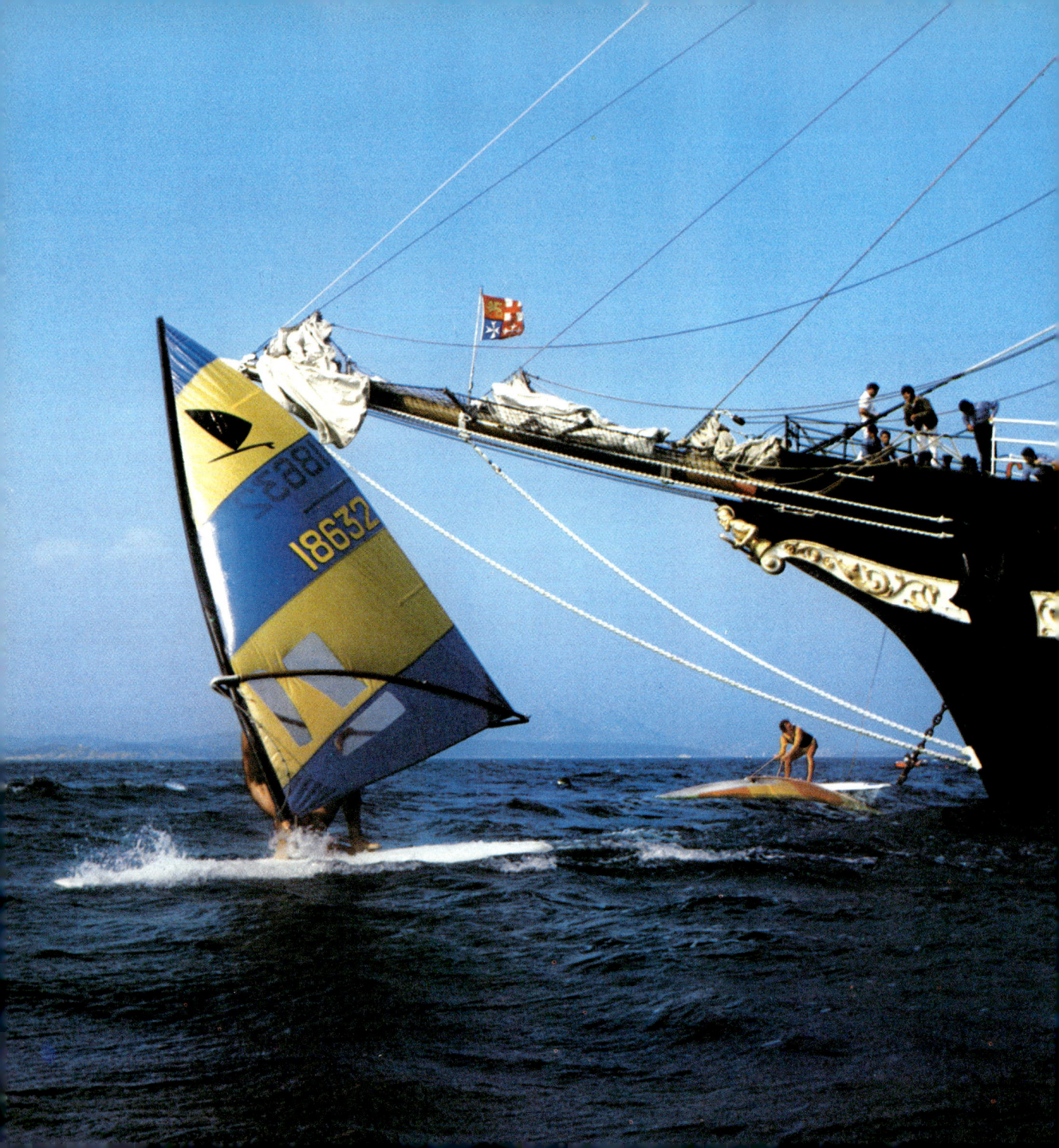

Windsurfing theory

Leafing through this book, you will certainly have noticed that the theory of windsurfing takes up more space here than in other books on windsurfing. A knowledge of the theory behind windsurfing is increasingly important as the sport becomes more and more sophisticated. A few examples will demonstrate this very clearly:

● Today, the windsurfing market is flooded with so many different makes of surfboard that you would be wise to study the subject in some detail before entering a windsurfing shop to buy a board.

● Particularly with the high-quality equipment now available, make sure you should make the best use of its advantages. Some background knowledge is a great help in this respect.

● At a time when suitable places for surfing are becoming more and more crowded, you must also develop a strong sense of responsibility for yourself and others afloat. To do this, you must be able to judge the weather, you must know the tides and other currents and you must be familiar with the Rules of the Road. Whilst there are only a few which operate between one sailboard and another, there are many which you should at least know. These are explained later in this book.

In any case, as you will appreciate, grappling with the theory behind windsurfing is an indispensable step towards getting to master more advanced techniques.

You will have also have noticed that the sections on the weather and the tides are quite long. This is because, as the developing surfboards begin to return to their sources in surfriding, i.e. the funboards, many windsurfers are attracted to coastal sailing. An ever-growing number of windsurfers want to put their sailing abilities to the test on the sea as well. They should all be aware of the dangers they might encounter. Misinterpreting weather changes and currents may only result in a few anxious minutes on a lake or a river, but at sea may well endanger the windsurfer's life. So one of the main objects of this section is a sound knowledge of the weather and the tides.

So that the theory does not become too tedious to read, every so often we have included some marvellous photos of extreme windsurfers in action. These photos

Games which would be dangerous and prohibited if the ship was under way.

will give you an idea of what windsurfing can mean. However, only a very, very few windsurfers are capable of sailing in such an extreme way. Do not get lured into such foolhardy adventures, however fit you may feel. No sensible skier would dream of skiing down the Matterhorn.

Boards and equipment

Although windsurfing is a very young sport, various generations of boards can already be distinguished, due to rapid developments in the manufacture of surfboards. Nevertheless, earlier types of board have not disappeared from the market and are still used. The different board ranges exist side by side, and rightly so; they allow for the different requirements and demands of the windsurfer.

In the next few pages we will discuss types of board.

Types of board
The allround/flatboard. The first board to be developed was the allround board or flatboard. Its appearance has much in common with the older type of surf boards, but its handling characteristics are determined by the same requirements as sailing boats. Daggerboard and mast foot well are so integrated into the board that the sailor's needs and expectations are met, e.g. good head up when tacking. What makes it outstanding is its versatility:

● you can use it successfully at regattas
● you can take part in freestyle events with it
● you can use it in the surf, albeit to a very restricted degree.

Even the first generation allround boards were able to hold the interest of many sportsmen for a long time. But very soon special demands began to be made on the equipment, due to the improved windsurfing skills of the sailors and their more sophisticated requirements. Thus, essentially, two new types of boards evolved:

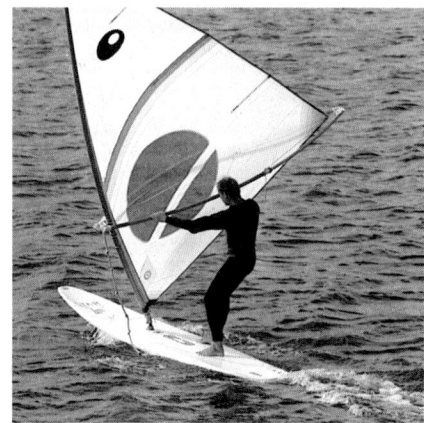

The picture shows an allround board with the original rig as supplied

● *Roundboards*, which have sailing characteristics very similar to a dinghy.
● *Strong wind/Funboards*, whose design concentrates more on the surfriding characteristics of the boards.

Roundboards. You would be justified in regarding a roundboard as a small sailing dinghy which can be steered like a surfboard. In profile it is similar to a dinghy. The tapering, turned up nose is very deep and changes towards the middle into a round underwater body, which ends in a wide, flat stern. A roundboard has a volume of 300 litres, 30% greater than that of an allround board. Because of its shape, it is faster than all other boards in weak and medium winds. When tacking, it ensures an optimum head up. However, the shape of its hull makes it very

Two roundboards in a regatta. The round hull is clearly visible ▼

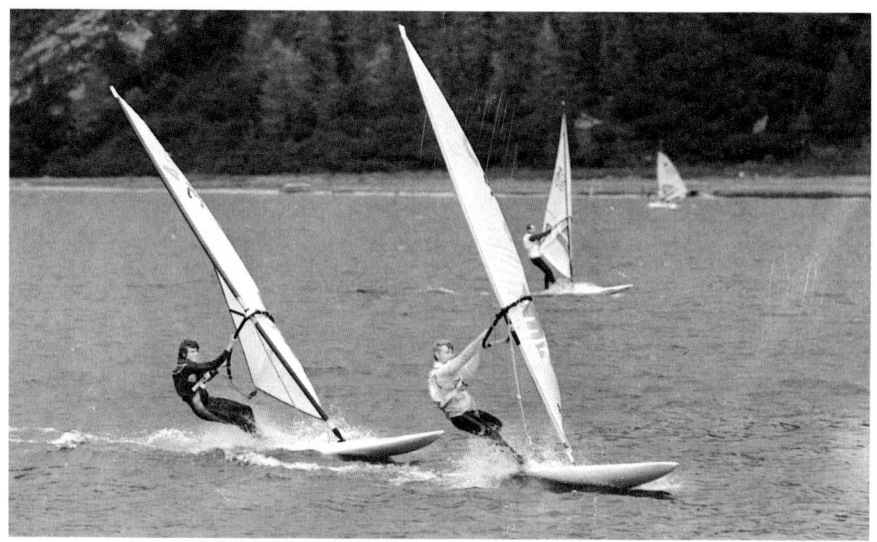

unstable, so only very experienced sailors can take to the water with it.

Funboards are more suitable for surfriding. They run lower in the water than allround boards, or even roundboards. On the other hand they are faster and more manoeuvrable in the planing phase. Their volume is reduced to the minimum to cut down board weight. The lack of buoyancy is compensated for by the dynamic drive of the sailing speed. Therefore, most funboards only have very bad sailing characteristics when the wind is below Force 4 and the board has not yet started to plane. If, however, the wind is strong enough, boards will increase their speed enormously after breaking through the displacement barrier.

Besides a low volume and a length of less than 3.5 m, funboards are characterised by their lightness (they only weigh between 10 and 15 kg) and by their flat hull. On most funboards the daggerboard is replaced by a larger or several smaller fins. For steering with your feet and jumping they are equipped with footstraps.

The most extreme forms of funboards evolved from the requirements of windsurfers in the waves off Hawaii. These boards are called *sinkers* or *semi-floaters*. They are between 2.10 and 2.80 m long, and their volume is less than 120 litres. They are faster and easier to manoeuvre than all other funboards. Due to their design features and the fact that they only perform really well in strong winds, funboards are recommended only for the real experts.

Karl Messmer on a sinker

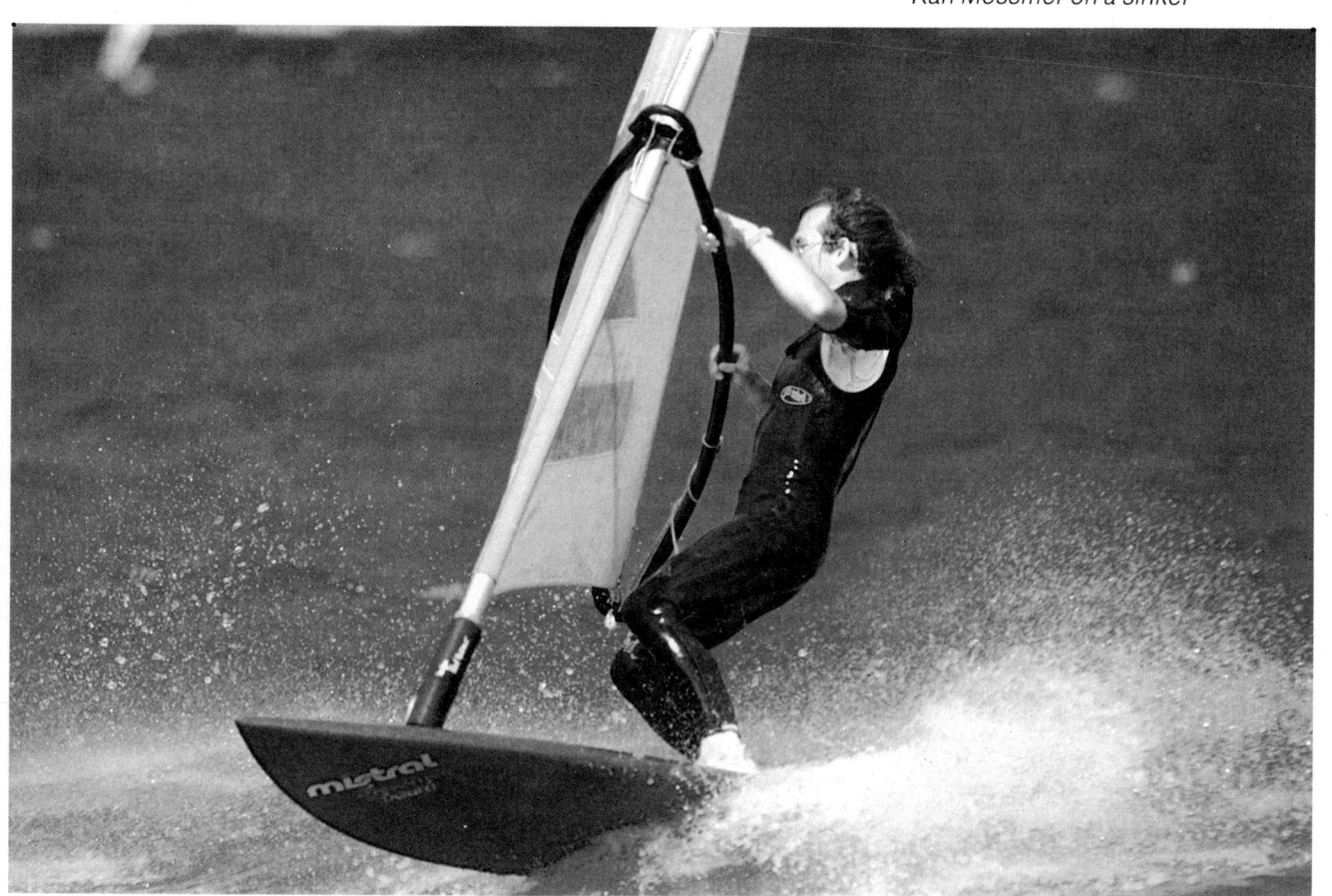

Allround funboards will sooner or later replace allround boards, for they share all the same characteristics and in addition they make it possible to get in on funboard surfing.

Allround funboards have a maximum length of 3.70 m and they have flat hulls. By using storm daggerboards which can be retracted flush with the bottom, or sickle-shaped daggerboards which can be reduced to fin size, the boards can be controlled by moving your weight inboard or out-board.

The tandem. The most sociable form of windsurfing. A tandem is operated by two sailors, with two rigs. The board is controlled by sheeting the forward or aft sail.

At one time, tandems achieved the highest speeds, but in strong winds, funboards are now much faster.

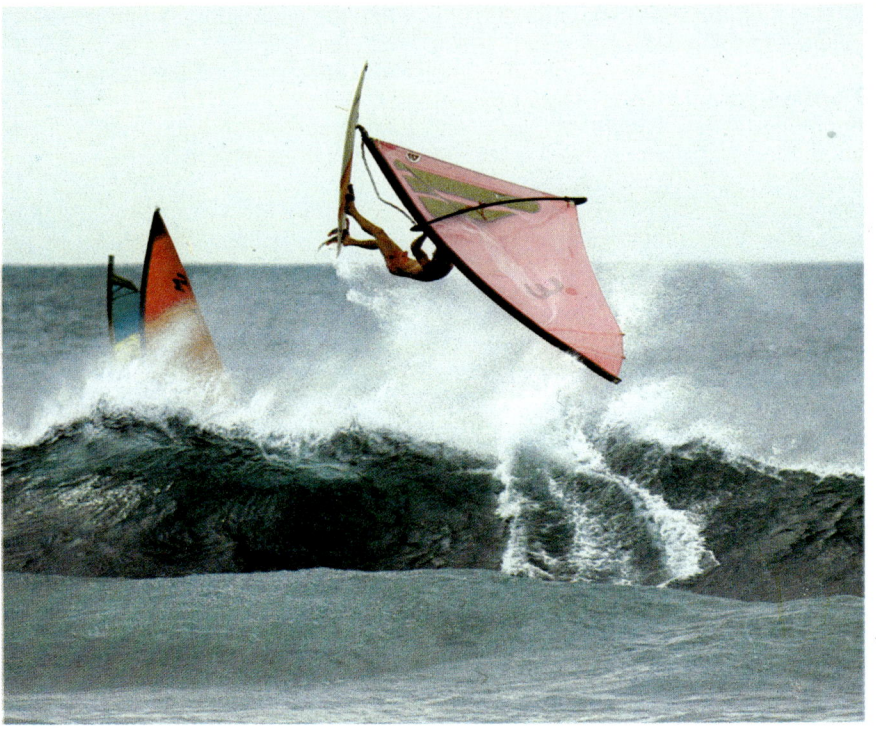

Tips for buying a board

It is a commonplace that somebody who does not know exactly what he or she wants will be lucky to get what he or she really needs. When buying a board, you are very likely to be unlucky unless you know what you want, because of the variety of boards offered.

Therefore we suggest that you ask yourself the following questions before entering a surfing shop.

● How much do you want to spend on your surfing equipment?
● How do you want to use your board? Do you want to sail in races or freestyle? Do you want to speed along, skimming over the water?
● Do you intend to sail in shallow waters or at sea?
● In what winds do you want to sail? Force 1–3, 3–6, 5 or more?
● How much sailing experience do you have? Are you a beginner, an advanced or an experienced sailor?
● How carefully are you going to handle your board? Do you need a robust board, or can you afford a more sensitive board?
● Which characteristics of a board are really important to you? Which ones can you do without?

What makes it so difficult to answer these questions is the fact that some of them are a matter of your own personal judgement. You should answer the questions about your experience honestly, because if you don't, you will spoil your fun in sailing by choosing the wrong board.

List all the characteristics your board is supposed to have, and mark them either dispensable or indispensable. You will certainly have to dispense with some characteristics in favour of others. A windsurfing board which combines all the advantages exists only in advertisements.

The design of a windsurfing board

Boards are made from fibre-reinforced duroplastics, i.e. synthetic resins such as epoxy and polyester resins, and from thermoplastics like polyethylene, ABS and ASA.

Thermosetting plastics possess a high degree of hardness and tensile strength, and are very light. By including fabrics in the synthetic resin, e.g. glass fibre, Kevlar, carbon fibre or mixed fabrics, the quality of thermo-setting plastics can be graded very finely.

Thermosetting plastics solidify only after the respective curing agents and accelerators have been added. After curing, their shape cannot be altered. It is relatively easy to prepare them, so they can also be processed by laymen.

Thermoplastics can only be processed with expensive equipment, which restricts their production to industrial manufacturers. They can be shaped by applying heat. Their shape can be altered again and again by repeated heating, and processing can continue.

ABS and ASA boards are moulded from sheets in a special process called deep drawing. Polyethylene boards are produced by roto-moulding and are blown, forming a plastic skin. If ABS and ASA boards are damaged, they can be repaired by a layman, provided the damage is only slight. Polyethylene boards can only be repaired with special hot-air welding equipment. Furthermore, they can only be joined by welding with polyethylene with the same molecular structure. ABS, like thermosetting plastics, can be mended with glass fibre-reinforced plastics or epoxy resin.

Because of their high tensile strength, thermoplastics are very resistant to damage by blows.

Almost all surfboards have a foam filling. This makes them more rigid, while at the same time remaining relatively light.

As a rule, *foamed polyurethane* and *polystyrene* are used. Custom made boards are manufactured from special white foams. The best known are Clark foam, Bennet foam, or the Australian phenolic foams. They are very hard and easy to cut and grind. After finishing, their smooth surface makes it possible to apply a transparent outer skin. This means that decorations or pictures can be sprayed on to the foam.

Types of construction. Besides the above-mentioned manufacturing methods with thermoplastics, glass fibre is also used for mass-producing surfboards. A mould release is applied to the negative mould of the board, which makes it possible to take the board out of the mould later. Then a gel coat is brushed into the mould to form a protective outer skin. When this has dried, layers of glass fibre soaked in resin are laid in place up to the desired wall thickness. Two moulds are made in this way — a top and a bottom half — which are glued together and filled with foam after curing.

Finishing a custom made board

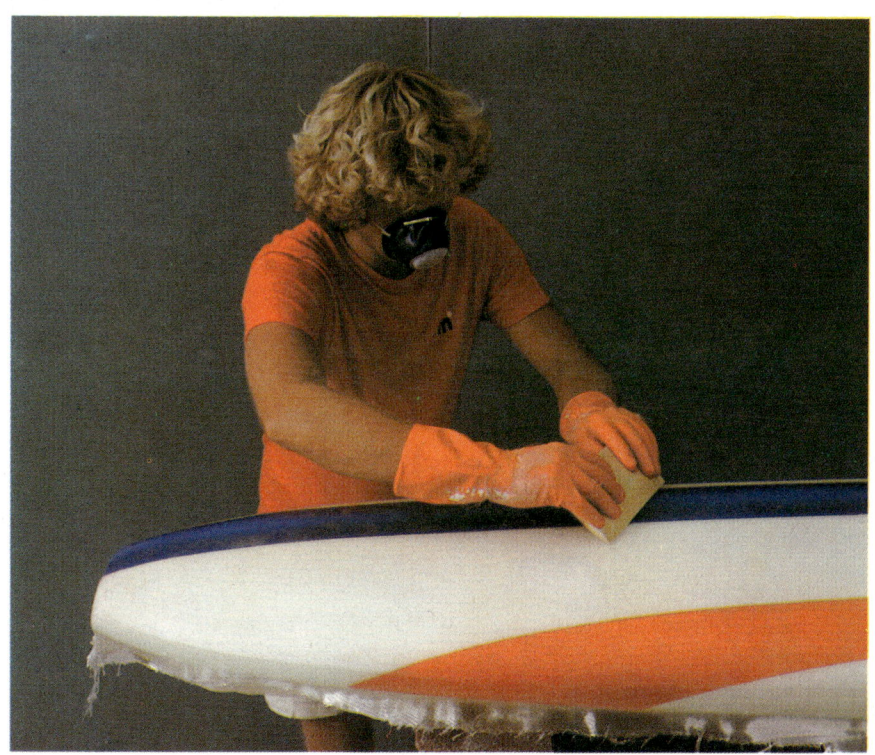

Custom made board construction is recommended for the home-made board: a foam block is shaped to the correct form and is enveloped with resin and fabrics.

The disadvantage of this method of construction is that it is very labour intensive and takes a long time. On the other hand each board is produced individually, so all possible details can be integrated into the board up to the last minute. This is one of the main reasons why board shapes have changed considerably since the introduction of the custom made board. Shapes have become more interesting and diverse.

For many years surfriding boards have been custom made. As a result, a variety of surfing terms has been adopted to refer to particular design features, such as the scoop, or different tail forms.

Sailboards are often named after their tail forms; the most common are pin, round, square, squash and fish tail (see illustration on page 63).

The forms give the boards different sailing characteristics — pin tails, for example, reach very high speeds, due to low friction in the gliding area. These boards allow extreme manoeuvres when riding the rail.

The following are the most important design features of boards.

A *rocker* is a curvature in the aft plane of a board, which makes the board faster. It also makes the board more manoeuvrable and it will more readily take off and jump.

Bevels are slight curvatures in the fore plane of the board. They permit the board to slide gently through the water, without sideslipping. This results in less drag when the bow submerges.

Modern boards are ground *concave* in the fore plane of the bow, in order to reduce the area which gets wet. This is because sideslipping is reduced by the air cushion in the concavity.

Scoop is the curvature at the nose of the board. At one time, scoops were curved up to 30 cm, if possible. At present normal boards are built with a moderate scoop (15 to 20 cm high).

Some manufacturers opt for *sandwich construction* to save weight and to increase the stiffness of the board. Sandwich construction means that foam or another filling is glued in between two skins. This results in a skin strength similar to that of a completely foamed board. However, the board is substantially lighter.

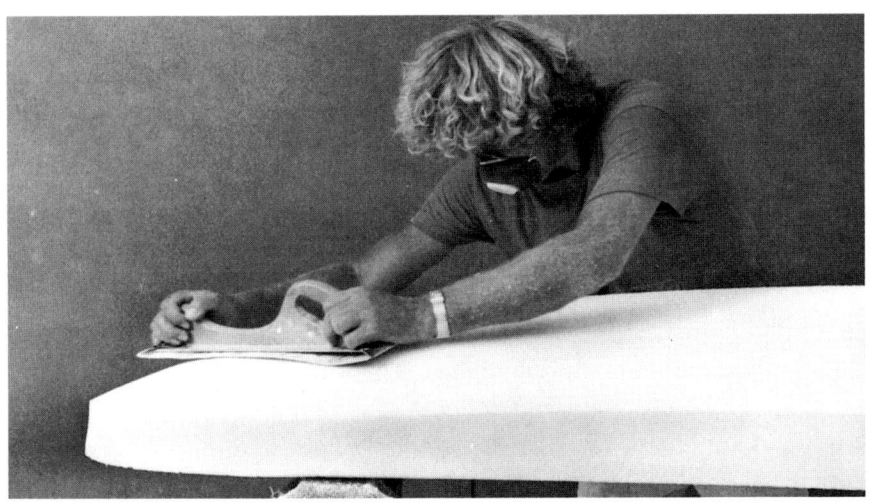

Shaping a custom made board ▲   *Two finished custom made boards* ▼

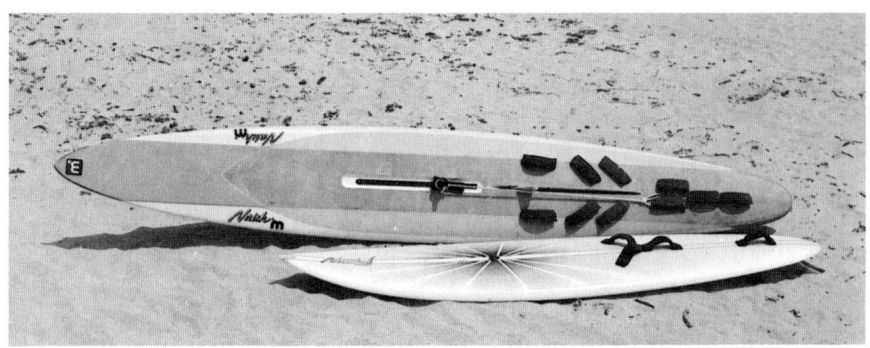

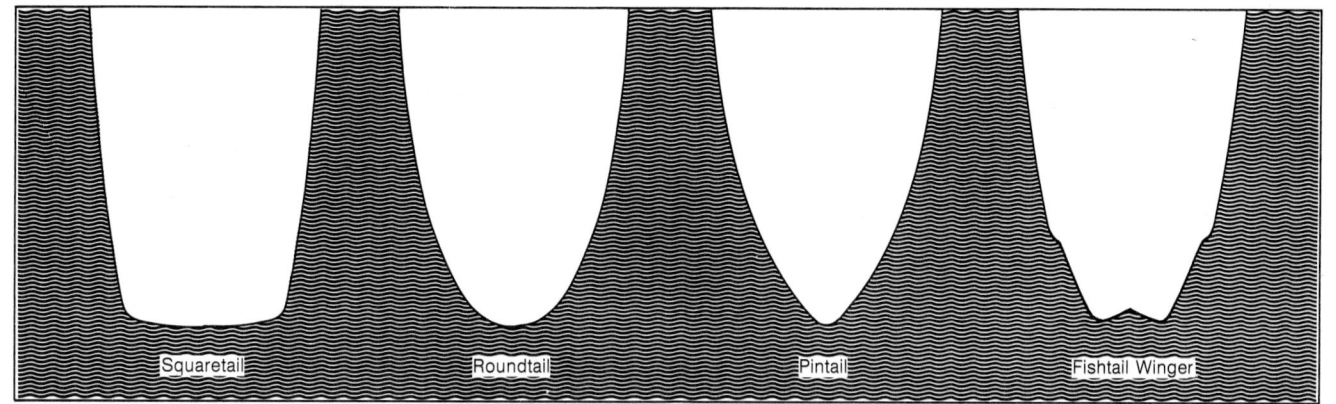

Squaretail   Roundtail   Pintail   Fishtail Winger

The parts of a sailing board

Daggerboards are made in many forms and from many materials, like laminated ply, glass fibre and polypropylene. The forms differ depending on how the board is used. Rigid straight daggerboards are used in regattas (65 to 70 cm long); storm daggerboards are smaller and shorter, the daggerboard area being moved aft. Most boards have retracting daggerboards, which can be either retracted completely flush with the bottom or swivelled aft.

    Since a large daggerboard area is exposed to water flowing along when the board cuts through the water, it is important to try and reduce the drag as much as possible. This is achieved by an optimum hydrodynamic form, which resembles the section of an airplane wing. Its exact shape, however, depends on the speed with which the section is required to cut through the water. It must be so shaped that the water flows along to the trailing edge with as little turbulence as possible.

    The shape of daggerboard most appropriate for you depends upon the speeds you wish, or are able, to

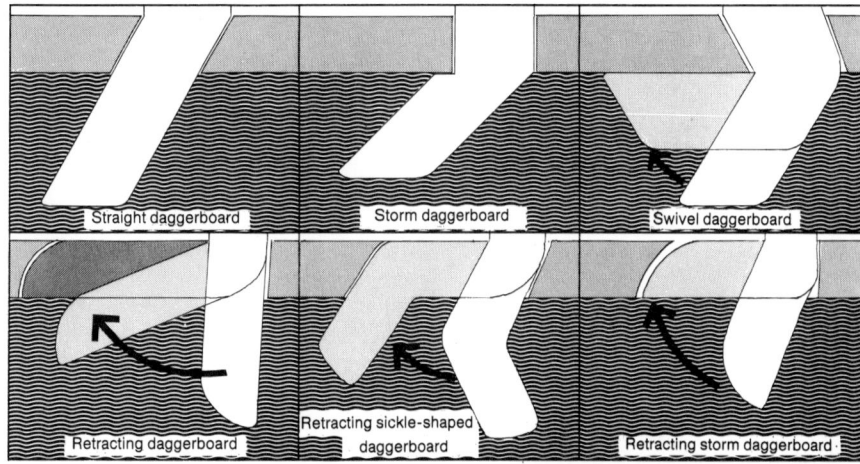

Straight daggerboard   Storm daggerboard   Swivel daggerboard

Retracting daggerboard   Retracting sickle-shaped daggerboard   Retracting storm daggerboard

achieve. A profile with a length (l) to thickness (t) ratio of 5:1 is appropriate for lower speeds: if you want to go more quickly a length to thickness ratio of 10:1 is more suitable. The thickest section of the board is about halfway along. The nose radius, i.e. the radius of a circle inscribed in the front part of the section, should be ⅕ of the thickest section. Optimum aft inclination of a section is 60 to 70°. You often read that the section must taper to a point. But in this case the water flow is not in contact with the section so

Characteristics of a flow section

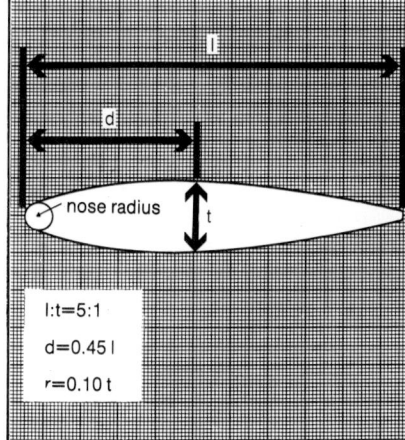

nose radius

l:t=5:1
d=0.45 l
r=0.10 t

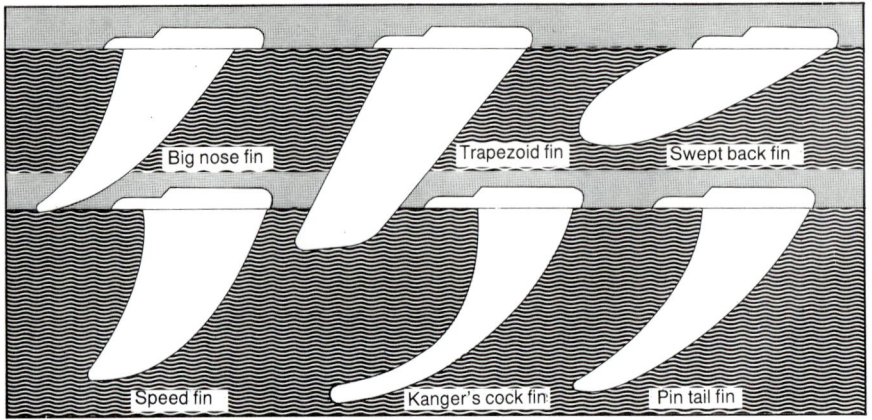

Big nose fin · Trapezoid fin · Swept back fin

Speed fin · Kanger's cock fin · Pin tail fin

The sail. The corners of the sail are called the *head*, (i.e. the top of the sail), the *tack*, (i.e. the corner down by the universal joint), and the *clew*, (i.e. the outer corner which is attached to the end of the wishbone).

A sail has three edges, which are called the luff, leech and foot. The luff is the edge of the sail between the head and the tack. The leech is the edge of the sail between the head and the clew. The foot is the bottom edge of the sail. The leech is supported by *battens* inserted in pockets.

Each sail must have a large enough window at the correct height, so that you have a clear view of the others on the water around you.

Clew and tack are each pierced with eyelets, through which the trim lines of the sails are passed (i.e. the downhaul and outhaul lines). A further, though minor, means of trimming the sail is provided by the size of the gap in the mast sleeve for the wishbone: the higher the wishbone is placed, the more the leech will be stretched, while the foot is loosened.

Surfing sails are made from Dacron and Mylar cloth. Mylar is a very expensive material which is sealed by a coat of plastic. It offers many advantages over Dacron, principally the optimum conversion of wind energy, because it hardly stretches or twists. As it is completely plastic sealed, no air can pass through, nor can water get into it. Thus Mylar cloth increases the speed of windsurfers by approximately 20 per cent as compared to Dacron. However, Dacron will last longer, because Mylar is more prone to V-shaped

that the trailing edge is in the turbulent area and extreme tapering will bring no advantages.

The fin. Like the daggerboard, the development of the fin was neglected for a long time; only after high speeds began to be achieved on funboards did the design and construction of fins begin to attract attention. Their task of stabilising direction was extended to stabilising lateral forces. The fin became ever larger, thus assuming the function of the daggerboard. On funboards the fin even replaced the daggerboard.

The illustration shows some fin forms.

Big nose and *speed fins* are standard fins for surfboards. With them, it is possible to sail at high speeds. Because of their form, they are very stable and allow radical manoeuvres. But they will tend to cause spinout (i.e. the board slides away due to turbulence from the fin at high speeds) if the surfer makes mistakes.

The regatta board is usually fitted with a *trapezoid fin*. Its form is almost ideal: a trapezoid fin with a good profile will have the most favourable water flow coefficient. It

will put very strong pressure on the fin case.

Kanger's cock and *pin tail* fins do not allow high speeds, because of their unfavourable flow pattern. On the other hand, they are not prone to spin out. However, they break easily because the area where they are attached to the board is small in relation to their length.

The *swept back fin* is suitable for shallow waters. It is also slow and prevents spinouts. It is subject to very high torsion forces, which means that it puts the quality of fin cases to the test.

Fins are made from glass fibre, Lexan, and wood.

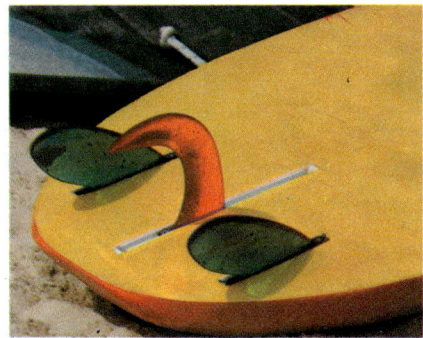

An adventurous combination of Kanger's cock and swept back fins

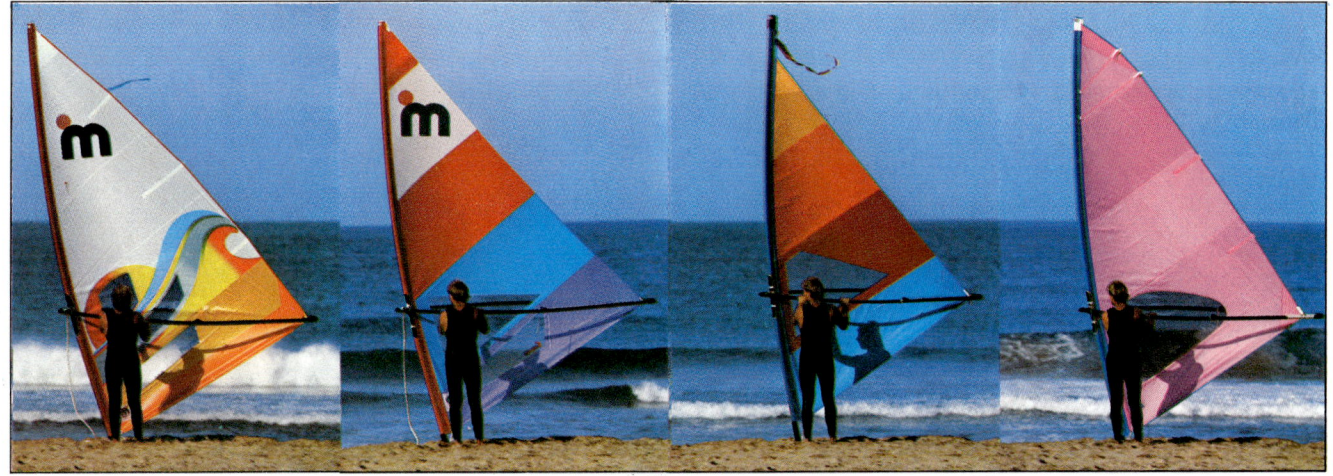

1

2

3

4

1 regatta sail
2 luxury sail
3 strong wind sail
4 fathead sail
Because sails 3 and 4 have a high clew, the mast stands upright when the wishbone is in a horizontal position.

cracks. Small cracks in the sail will very soon widen into large holes.

Types of sail. As the illustrations on the facing page show, two types of sail exist: sails for allround and regatta boards (1 and 2) and sails for faster boards (3 and 4).

Equipping a funboard with an allround board sail entails obvious disadvantages: with a low clew, the wishbone will often slide through the sea at high speeds.

There are also disadvantages when an allround board is equipped with a funboard rig. The drive of the sail is caused by the lift, i.e. the difference in pressure between the leeward and windward sides of the sail. The greater the difference in pressure, the stronger will be the force of the wind on the sail.

Tips for buying a sail

As is the case with buying the rest of the windsurfing equipment, you should have certain points in mind when you buy a sail.

● The price you want to pay.
● How you will use the sail.
● The rigidity of your mast.
● The length of your wishbone.

Before you buy you should check the quality of the cloth:

● Take hold of the cloth with both hands, and press your thumb (though not your thumbnail) into the cloth. Insufficiently tempered cloth will retain the thumb impression. You should refrain from buying sails made of such cloth, even if they are cheaper.

A further criterion is the workmanship of the sail.

● Check the seams.
● The corners must be reinforced several times.
● The eyelets in tack and clew must fit tightly.
● The cloth round the window must not have creases.

All other points can only be checked with the correctly trimmed sail heeled into the wind:

● Try to measure the profile. (Where is the deepest point in the curvature of the sail? Does the sail crease?) The profile can be measured by looking at the curvature of the seams. Often, coloured lines printed on the sail will reveal its curvature.
● Check whether the window is large enough for you to have a good view around, and make sure the window is placed high enough.
● The position of the gap in the mast sleeve for the wishbone must be at least as high up as your shoulders. There should still be space above it. Its edges must be reinforced.

Attempts are made to keep the gap between foot and board as small as possible, to avoid air flows which equalise the pressure on the sail. With a high clew or fathead sail on an allround board, the gap between foot and board is very wide, with the pressure being equalised from the foot upwards.

The mast foot. The mast foot too has undergone development. From a T-piece made of wood or metal loosely fitted into the board has evolved a sophisticated safety mast foot.

Safety mast foot. Previously, whenever the sailor wanted to sheet in with a slightly canted board, the mast foot came loose from the mast foot well. When you pulled the wishbone upwards to keep balance, rig and board were separated. Only experts were then able to avoid a fall. Very soon mast feet were wrapped with insulating tape and rammed into the board. Now they never came loose at all. This resulted in crushed feet, trapped between mast and board.

Then Mistral put on the market the first mast foot system that was to a certain extent adjustable. The mast foot was fixed in the mast foot well by means of a metal clamp, which released the mast foot at low or high loads, depending on how much it had been bent.

Subsequently, release devices have been developed which can be adjusted very precisely. The most frequently used system consists of a mast foot which will compress a rubber hose by means of a gland. When the gland is tightened along the corresponding thread, the rubber is compressed longitudinally. The rubber hose thickens as a result

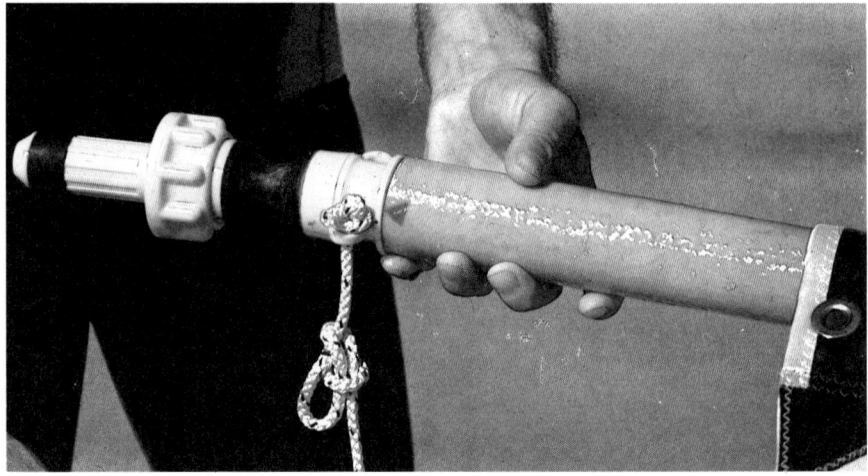

and becomes wedged in the mast foot well.

The mast foot/universal joint.

There are two different ways of providing the rig with the mobility which is necessary for steering.

These are the *universal joint* (UJ), and the *rubber joint*, which was originally used for engine suspension in the automotive industry.

Make sure the mast foot joint is firm. Soft joints complicate accurate steering and will warp under stress. Moreover, they are a safety risk, because they break more easily. The metal plates at the end must be vulcanised in to prevent them from tearing off.

The mast. The materials used for making masts, like those for making boards, are polyester or epoxy, glass fibre, carbon fibre, Kevlar or composite textures. In addition, Duralumin is used.

Make sure that the mast is sealed at both ends to prevent water from getting in. It should also be

The safety mast foot with rubber joint and downhaul line. The rubber on the mast foot journal is held apart by a screw to wedge the journal in the board

reinforced where the wishbone is attached to it.

There are on the market masts with differing degrees of rigidity. When buying a mast, you should see to it that the rigidity of the mast matches the fullness of the sail. A sail will only provide optimum drive when it has been correctly matched with the mast.

Inexperienced surfers are advised not to buy a combination of rigid mast and sail. This combination will give an optimum conversion of wind energy into speed, but will not cushion sudden gusty winds. As a consequence, a surfer with a bad technique will soon become tired.

A further point to consider is the weight and the diameter of the mast. When buying glass fibre masts, transparent ones are recommended. They will reveal at a very early stage the hair-line cracks that will eventually result in a rupture.

Wishbones are made from aluminium and covered in rubber for heat insulation and grip.

The main differences between various types of wishbone are in their length, diameter, the form of the tube and their weight.

The fore boom end fittings of all wishbones are padded. Thus the board is protected from damage which may occur after catapult falls when the rig hits the board.

The wishbone must be long enough to allow the sail to be trimmed fully. However, it should not be too long. If the distance between clew and the aft boom end fitting is too long, the clew is not sufficiently fixed, and the centre of effort (CE) changes its position in the sail.

The wishbone should be fairly slim, which will make it easier to handle and control of the rig more precise. If you want to surf in stronger winds, you should use a stiffer wishbone. The decisive factor is the degree of stiffness of the aluminium and the strength of the boom end fittings. Soft wishbones will stretch when under strain. As a consequence the form of the sail will change and the Centre of Effort (CE) will move.

Important accessories. Each sailboard must be provided with a safety device for securing the rig if the mast foot slips out. This safety device corresponds to the ski strap: if the mast foot comes out of the board, the rig safety line keeps board and rig connected together. Modern sailboards include a safety rope which operates from the bow. It will also resist waves. A strong

rubber shockcord is fixed on the bow. This cord is guided through a channel to the mast foot and is fastened there. Because of its elasticity strong currents, such as occur in surf waves, cannot tear the cord, and the board can run with the current and the breaking wave.

Each surfboard must have a *towing eye*, which is integrated into the nose of the board and which can be used for towing the board away.

Useful accessories. For sails with a long luff, a *mast extension* is required, which is inserted between the base of the mast and the mast foot.

Footstraps are required for precise control of funboards with your feet. Frequently you will see boards with 10 to 12 footstraps mounted on them. You should only mount the number of footstraps you really need. Bear in mind that too

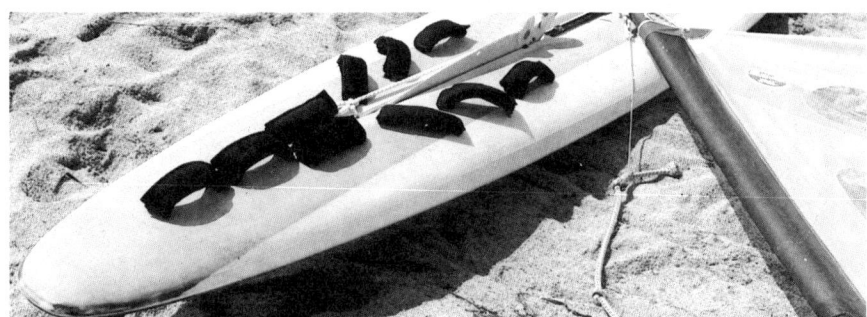

Beware of tripping over footstraps! In many sailing positions too many footstraps are annoying. Only fit the number you really need

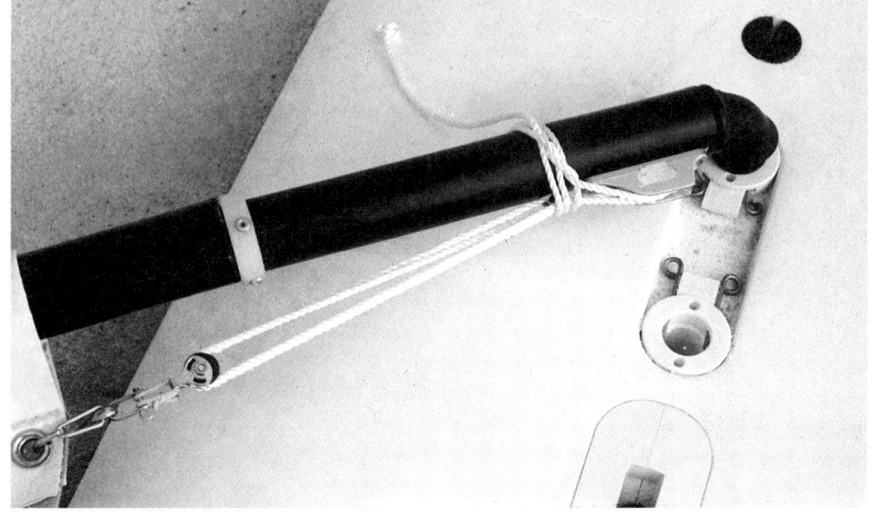

Mast extensions are used for sails with a long luff. Using this extension, the window can be adjusted correctly to your eye level and the clew can be lifted further up, to prevent it from dragging through the water

many straps will get in the way when you need to change position on the board and that you need none at all in certain sailing positions.

If you want to save yourself the effort of belaying the downhaul line to the mast extension, attach a compressor, unless there already is one built-in, to grip the downhaul line (see illustration on page 67).

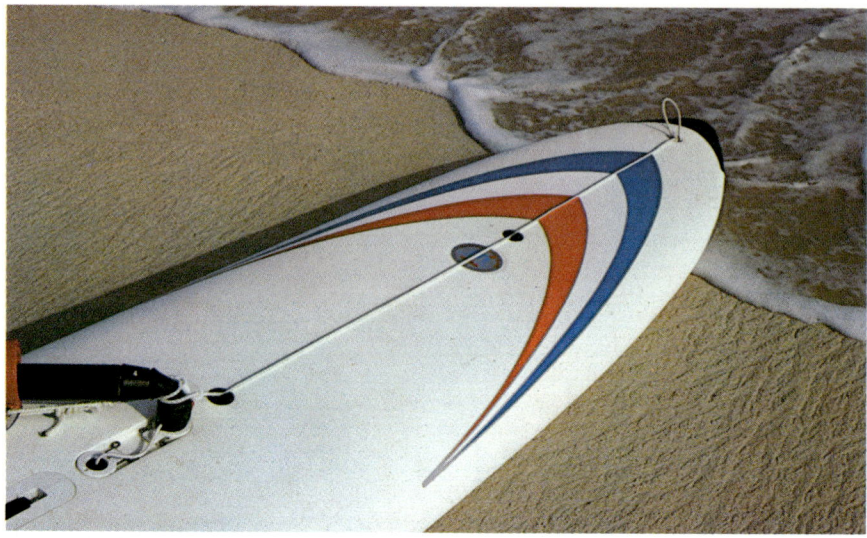

A modern rig safety rope runs from the bow to the mast foot

This Hawaiian uphaul is too short, and wastes some of the strength which is needed for pulling up the rig ▼

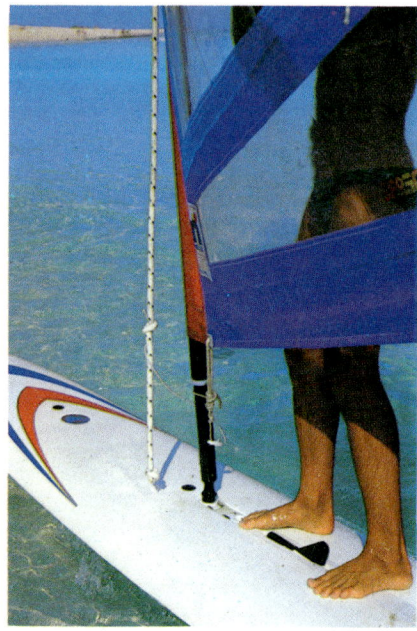

With its knots the uphaul rope reaches down to the board

Most *uphaul ropes* supplied with mass-produced boards are too thin and too short for pulling up the rig correctly. You should immediately replace them with a proper rope. The uphaul rope with its knots should reach down to the mast foot so that you can pull the rig out of the water by keeping your back straight and by leaning backwards slightly (page 18).

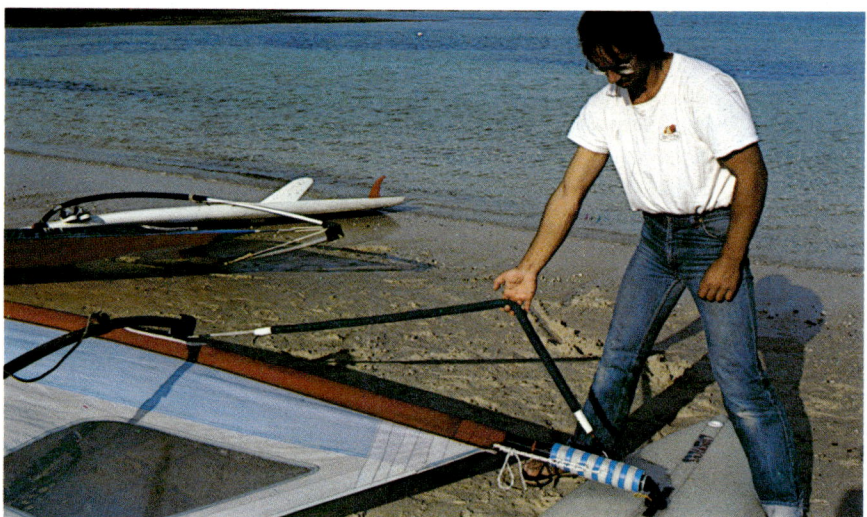

Avoid older Hawaiian uphauls: they make pulling up the rig very hard work.

It is advisable to use modern uphaul ropes which are tied rigidly like conventional ropes, but consist of several individual ropes tied together loosely. In this way, they afford a good grip like the old Hawaiian uphauls, but use the uphaul forces much more effectively.

Clothing

Windsurfing suits are made from neoprene, Rubatex, Yamato-neoprene or polyurethane. The interior is lined with cloth. Since they are very prone to tearing, their outer side is frequently bonded with other materials for protection.

When you buy a windsurfing suit, you should think about the following aspects in advance:

● How much money do you want to spend?
● What stresses will the suit be subjected to when in use and transported?
● What temperatures is it supposed to protect you against?

In addition, check the strength and elasticity of the material. As a rule, double-bonded suits are less elastic than single-bonded ones. The softest materials are Rubatex and Yamato-neoprene.

Single-bonded suits retain heat best, because the water drains off them and cannot take heat from the body by evaporation.

The fit of a suit is determined by the material and the cut. Fit is particularly important round the arms and in the crotch. The material round the arms, especially on the lower arm, must be so elastic that the blood circulation is not restricted. For this reason, some new suit types have arms made from a cloth-like material, e.g. Goretex.

If you wish to surf in cold weather, you should buy a *dry suit*. Most dry suits are made from waterproof plastics with thin rubber seals at the arms, feet and neck. They do not provide warmth themselves, but you can wear a track suit or thermal underwear underneath. Make sure that the suit is made from a material which is waterproof, but lets your skin breathe, so that you really keep dry in your dry suit. Otherwise, sweat will condense and collect between your shoulder blades and your body will get colder and colder.

Shoes are an essential part of your windsurfing clothing. They protect your feet against injuries from sharp stones and broken glass. In the beginning, simple non-slip plimsolls will do. You would be advised to wear them together with neoprene socks to prevent blisters and improve heat insulation.

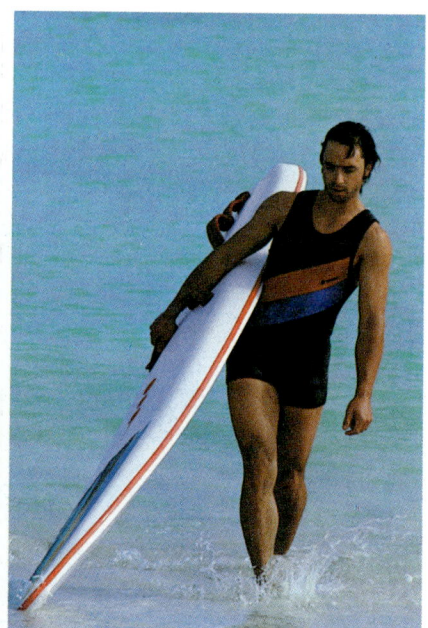

For warm days a shorty, which keeps your body warm, is useful

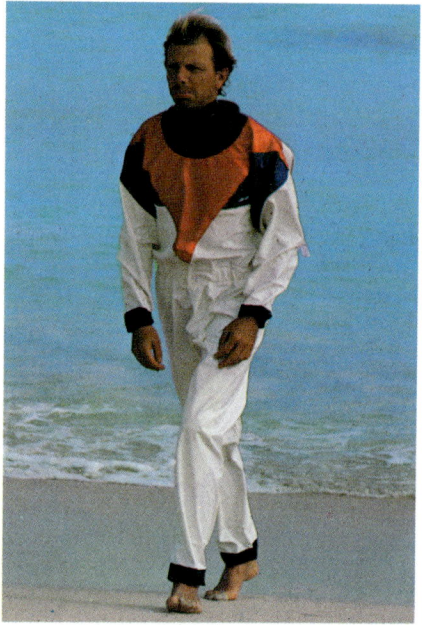

If you want to surf in winter, you should wear a dry suit

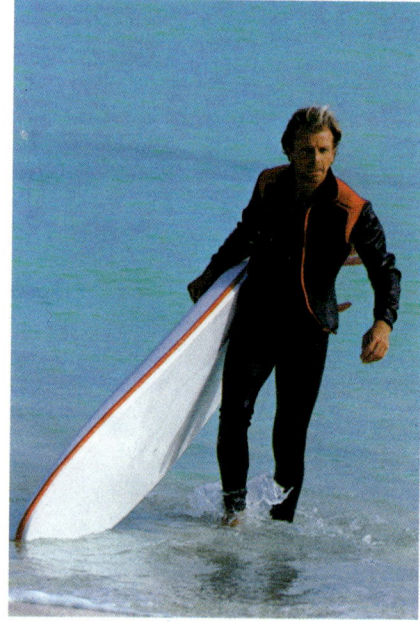

The long john with jacket

Sailing theory

Directions

The *port* side of the board is the left side as you look towards the bow. The right side is the *starboard* side.

When the wind is blowing on the port side, then you are on *port tack*. Conversely, when the wind blows over the starboard side, then you are on *starboard tack*.

The front end of the board is the *bow* and the back end is the *stern*. Objects which are in front of you are *ahead*. Things behind the board are *astern*.

Things on either side are described as *abeam* – "on the port beam" means on the left side of the board.

Right ahead or *right astern* refer to an object directly in front of or behind the board.

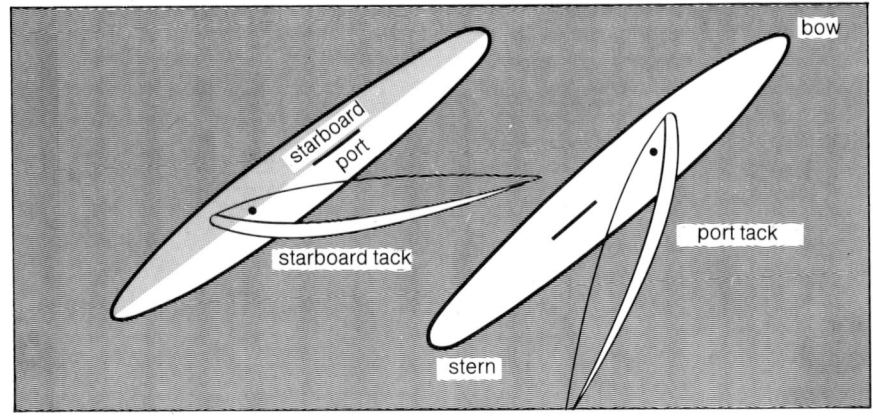

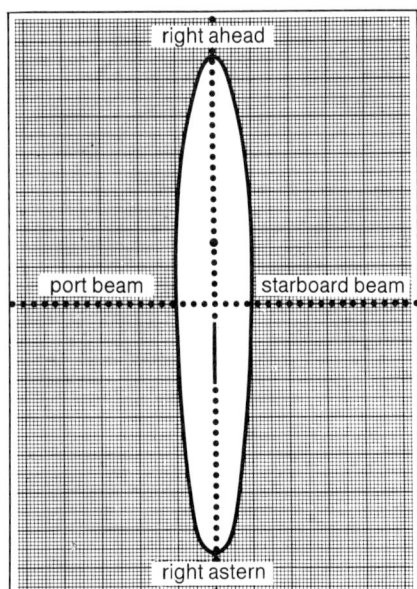

Windward refers to the side of an object which points towards the wind. *Leeward* refers to the side which is turned away from the wind.

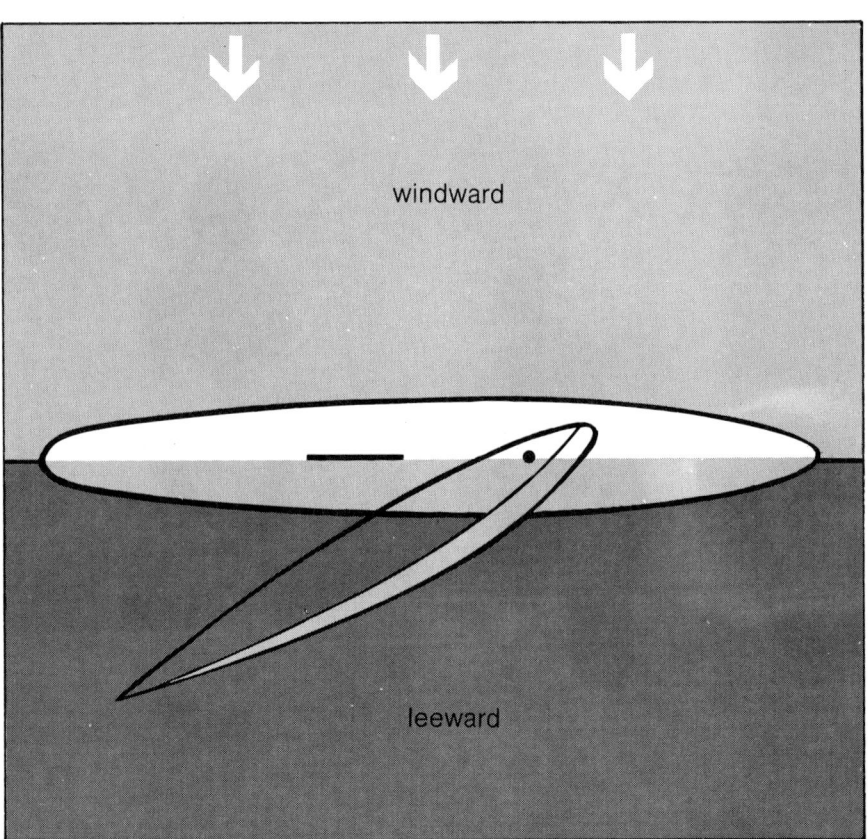

Changing directions and positioning the sail. All changes in course are described in relation to the direction of the wind. They are called
● *heading up*, which means changing a board's direction towards the wind, so that it is beating more
● *bearing away*, which means changing the board's direction away from the wind, so that it is heading away from the wind.
Tilting the rig back results in the board heading up. If you rake it forward it will bear away.
So, if you are sailing in a straight line and the board shows an inclination to head up, rake the rig forward and sheet in. If you don't, the board will go on heading up until the wind hits the leeward side of your sail which will push you over and into the water. The constant tendency is for the board to head up. As soon as you have corrected this tendency, set the rig straight up. You will find that these alterations are constantly necessary.

The direction in relation to the wind. The direction in which a board moves is called the *course*. Particular courses in relation to the wind are given special names, which apply as much to sailing as to windsurfing.
A beating course is when you sail as close as possible to the wind.
A beam reach is a course which runs exactly at right angles to the wind.
Running means going in exactly the same direction as the wind.
Courses at an angle to the wind are called *broad reaches*.
Sail-operated vessels are restricted in their movements when sailing against the wind. If they sail too close when sheeted in they will eventually go head to wind, stop sailing and drift backwards. When you feel you are slowing up like this, sheet out and bear away to pick up speed again. If that means that you are going in the wrong direction, then tack through the wind. Look at the circular diagram and you will be able to work out that the boats on the right-hand side of the picture are on the starboard tack and those on the left side of the picture are on port tack.

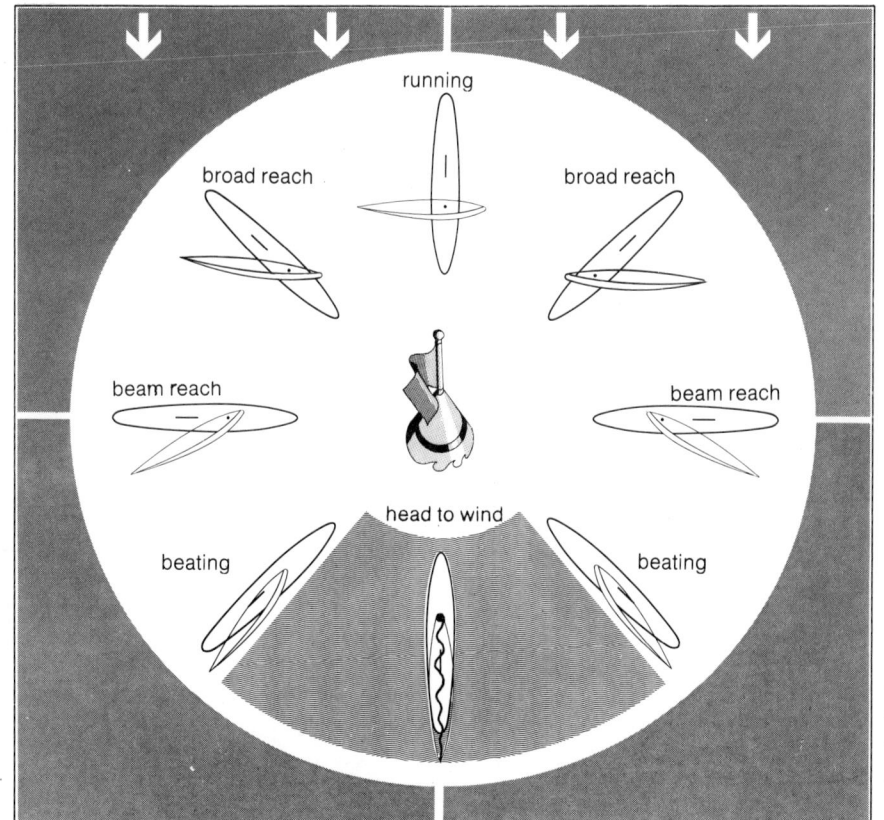

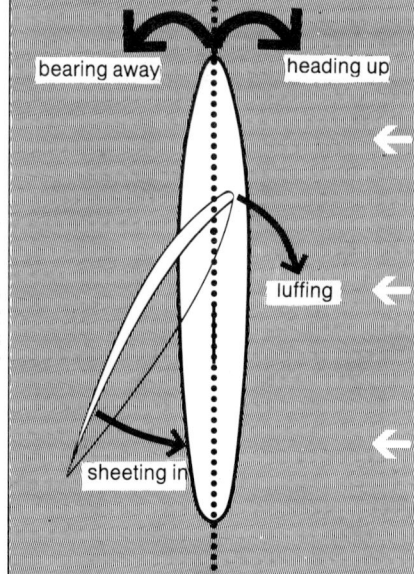

Wind propulsion

The propulsion of the board is governed by two different principles which act together but vary in their effects according to the course chosen.

The first of these can be seen most clearly in running courses. It is resistance sailing.

Resistance sailing. If the sail is luffed as far as possible it offers an area of resistance to the wind. When the wind acts on the sail, it causes the sail and board to move. The force thus produced increases linearly in proportion to the area of sail which is presented; in other words the more air is captured, the faster the board will go.

The second principle becomes apparent in courses at an angle or at right angles to the wind. This is lift sailing.

Lift sailing. The sail is placed at an angle of attack of approximately 20 degrees. This causes the air to be deflected from its straight line along the sail. The sail's camber reduces the distance the windward air particles have to move in comparison to the leeward air particles. Thus the leeward air accelerates, and the resulting force creates a suction towards leeward, which affects the whole area of the sail. The sum of all the forces may be imagined as acting on one point, the *Centre of Effort*. Here the forces seem to act at right angles to the chord of the sail.

The *total force* acts at an angle to the board. It is made up of two parts, the driving force and the leeway force. In order to obtain the best possible driving force, which in many courses is smaller than the leeway force, the leeway force

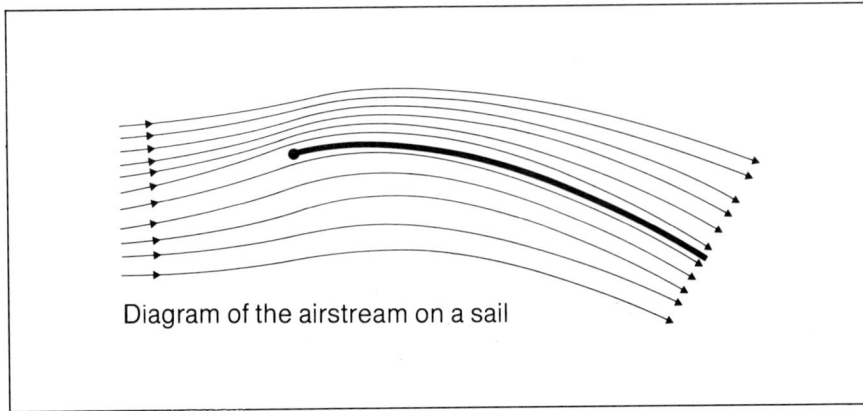

Diagram of the airstream on a sail

under the water must be counteracted by an opposite force. This is created by the daggerboard, which substantially enlarges the area of lateral resistance of the board. Although the daggerboard reduces the leeway force (i.e. the sideways displacement of the board when in motion), it can also bring about a capsize fall, as it acts below the centre of buoyancy.

The wind acts on the whole area of the sail, but the forces involved can be imagined as combining to act on one point.

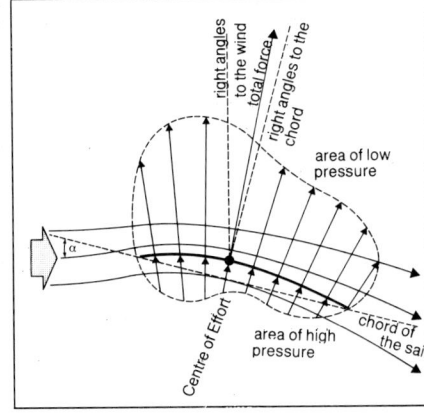

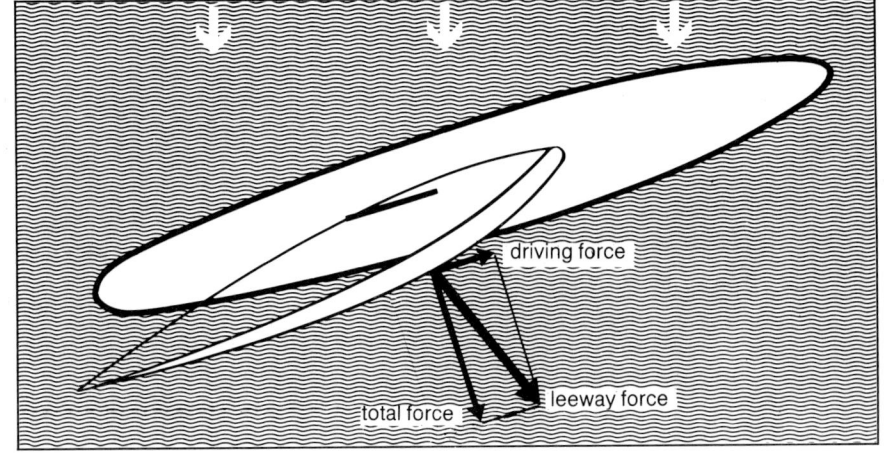

The leeway. Due to the large contribution made by the leeway force to the total force, the course steered in many cases does not correspond to the course which you actually sail. For this reason, beginners are often surprised to discover that while they are heading exactly towards a certain point, they are to leeward when they arrive. The distance between the point aimed at and the point actually reached corresponds to the *leeway*. It is related to the course and also to the speed of the board, as the resistance offered to the leeway force by the lateral view is dynamic. The faster a board goes, the smaller is its leeway.

The sailing wind. So far we have taken the wind to be uniform, but this needs to be qualified.

If you ring the Meteorological Office or determine the wind's direction with your sail you will find out in what direction the *real* or *true wind* is blowing. When you move through calms you can still feel a wind. It comes from directly ahead, increasing in strength as you move faster.

As you move forward on your board, the true wind combines with the wind caused by the movement of your board to produce a wind of yet another direction and speed. This is the *apparent wind*. It always blows at a greater angle than the true wind. Its strength and direction depend on the relative strength of the true wind and the wind due to the movement of the board. The faster a board is travelling, the more the apparent wind hauls forward. As the sail is always positioned in relation to the apparent wind, even very fast boards have their sail sheeted in for beam reach or broad

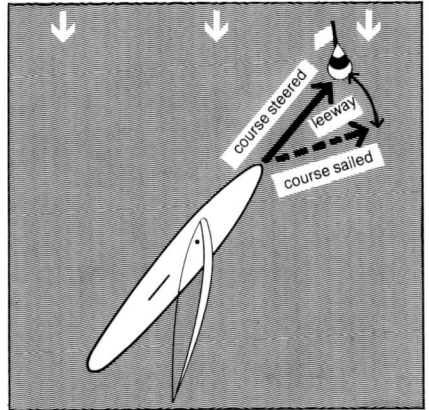

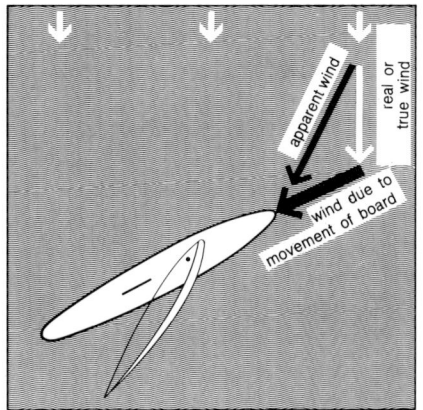

reach. The sail is luffed only when a running course is reached.

Especially in windsurfing, a good knowledge of the effects of the apparent wind is essential.

Surfing in gusty winds. In gusty winds, the apparent wind keeps changing direction: in a gust, it initially backs towards the direction of the true wind. If the board then moves faster, the apparent wind veers towards the bow again. So the

sail must first be luffed and then sheeted in again.

This method will make you lose headway when beating. We therefore recommend keeping the sail in position and heading up so as to maintain the ideal angle towards the wind. If you alternately head up and bear away at the right moment, you will be able not only to maintain your headway in gusty winds but even to increase it and with care you will not find yourself in a head-to-wind position.

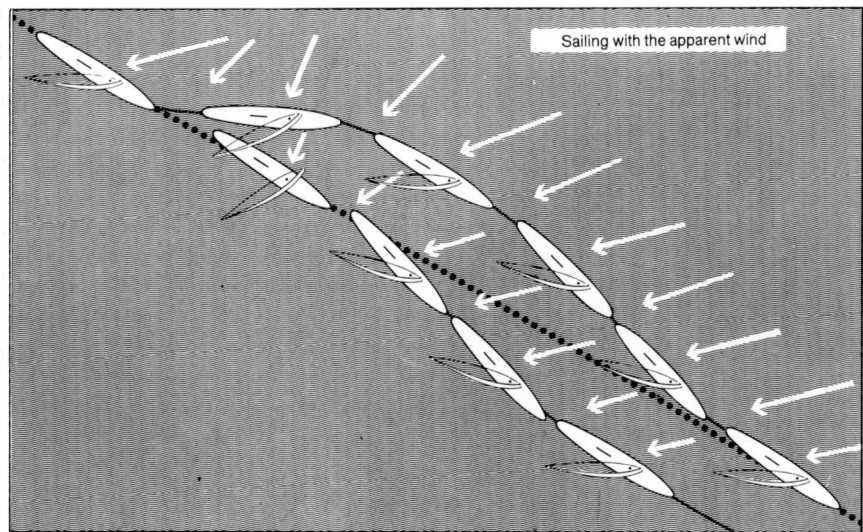

Sailing with the apparent wind

Surfing in strong winds. Anyone setting out in a strong wind may find that his sail suddenly comes flying at him even though he has started correctly. What has happened? A surfboard only takes a few yards to reach its maximum speed. As a consequence, the apparent wind jumps towards the bow immediately after the start. Any surfer who does not sheet in strongly in order to adjust to the probable wind direction will have the apparent wind coming at his sail from windward, causing him to fall into the water.

Surfing in waves. A surfboard is accelerated by the current in front of a wave. This causes the apparent wind to veer to the bow, so that you have to sheet in. The current behind a wave slows the board down and the apparent wind backs to the direction of the real wind. The sail has to be luffed.

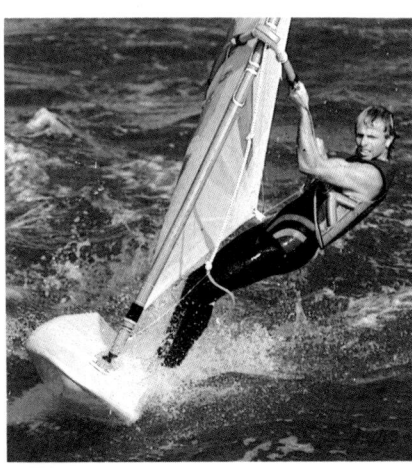

Travelling in small waves may be difficult. Whenever the wave passes you, you will find it difficult to luff in order to regain your balance and speed

Steering

The wind force acting on the Centre of Effort is opposed by the board's underwater resistance. Like the wind force, the forces of underwater resistance may also be imagined as combining in one point. In physics this is called the *Centre of Lateral Resistance*. A vertical line passing though this point forms the centre of rotation around which the board is steered. The force acting on the Centre of Lateral Resistance runs directly counter to the force of the wind. When the force of the wind and that of the water resistance are balanced in one line, the board goes straight ahead: it is *trimmed*.

When the force of the wind moves in relation to the centre of rotation, the board begins to turn. When the wind propulsion shifts to windward and towards the bow, the forces on the front end of the board become stronger, causing it to bear away.

When the wind propulsion is shifted to leeward and towards the tail, it acts on the stern. The bow, being situated in front of the centre of rotation, turns towards the wind, causing the board to head up (see top diagram on page 75).

Even while you are steering, you have to ensure that the sail is kept in the ideal position in relation to the wind. For this purpose, steering movements are initiated by tilting the rig parallel to the sail. If you move your rig in a different direction, you will either continue straight on, or, if there is a strong breeze, go into a catapult fall (see pages 28–29).

You can also shift the force of underwater resistance instead of that of the wind. If your board is equipped with a daggerboard, you can shift the Centre of Lateral Resistance to leeward and towards the tail in order to bear away. If if is shifted to windward or towards the bow, your board will head up.

Weather helm and lee helm

The terms weather and lee helm are taken from sailing. They refer to a boat's tendency to head to the wind or bear away if not corrected.

These terms must be defined differently for windsurfing. As the rig we have here is not restricted in its movements, and is used to steer and propel the board at the same time, weather helm is not the same as with sailing boats. On a boat, the mast is fixed rigidly and, depending on its position, the boat will, if not altered with the rudder, either go straight on (if it is in trim), or have a tendency to bear away (lee helm), or try to head up (weather helm).

With windsurfers such tendencies can be stopped immediately by tilting the rig in the appropriate manner. Thus the board can always be trimmed.

However, not every shift of the rig which is intended to trim the board will help it to make speed. So weather and lee helm must be defined as the board's tendency to head up or bear away with the rig in its normal position.

The methods of counteracting the weather and lee helm of a surfboard are not so straightforward as in the case of sailing boats. They depend, among other things, on the volume and the underwater shape of the board, and whether the lateral view is spread over the whole length of the board or centred in a large daggerboard plane. A funboard, for instance, with its skeg surface hardly larger than the whole of the rest of the lateral view together, has stronger weather helm when you

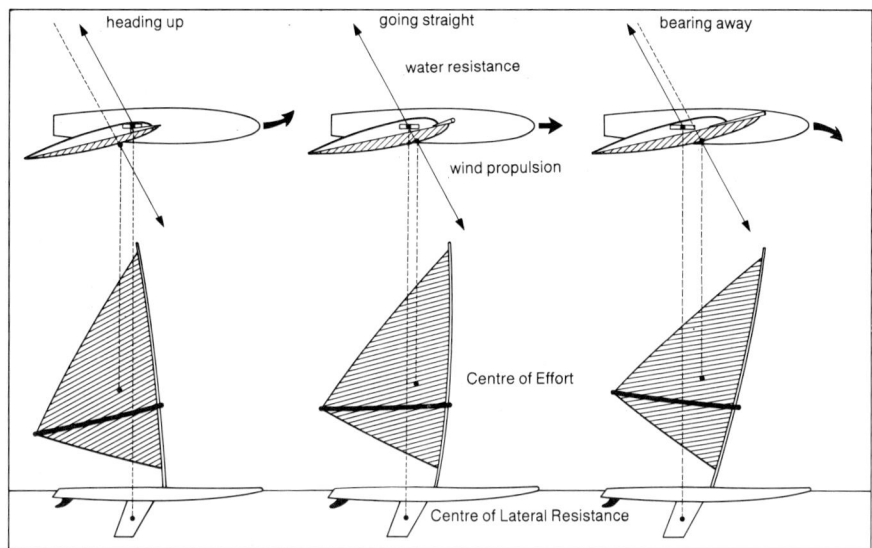

heading up   going straight   bearing away

water resistance

wind propulsion

Centre of Effort

Centre of Lateral Resistance

place the mastfoot further to the front. A roundboard with its daggerboard, on the other hand, will have more lee. The important thing with funboards is that the bow lies lower in the water, so that it plunges even deeper if the front mastfoot well is used. This causes the Centre of Lateral Resistance to move so far to the front that it creates a weather helm in the board. For roundboards the rig movement is more decisive. The Centre of Lateral Resistance hardly changes its position, as the forces of resistance are concentrated on the daggerboard anyway.

The interplay of water resistance and sailing force can be felt very clearly on the various types of boards when a gust comes up: initially, a funboard will rise on to its plane in the tail section. If you do not move the rig out of its position, the board bears away. When the gust dies down, the board is lowered from the plane and heads up.

With a daggerboard, however, a gust shifting the sailing force to the stern will cause the board to head up.

Displacing and planing

Any boat will produce waves as it moves through the water: a bow wave and a tail wave. Even boards have these if they are *displacement sailing*. The maximum speed is then dependent upon the speed of the wave. It is calculated as 1.6 times the square root of the length in feet of the board at the water-line, the result being measured in miles per hour. A real roundboard with a water-line length of, say, 14ft can have a maximum speed of 6mph ($\sqrt{14} \times 1.6 = 6$mph). All surfboards, including the roundboards, are capable of leaving this wave system and of moving far faster than the displacement barrier. For this reason, the rule "The longer the board, the faster it sails", which you can find in older books about windsurfing, is wrong for modern surfboards. A surfboard's speed is determined mainly by its ability to plane early and to waste a minimum of wind energy on counteracting forces produced by factors such as high board weight or excessive skin friction.

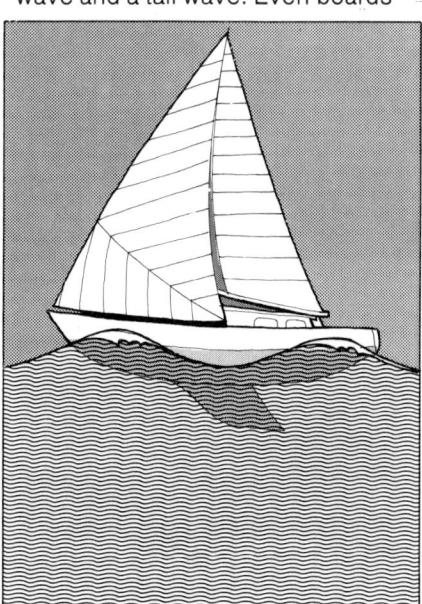

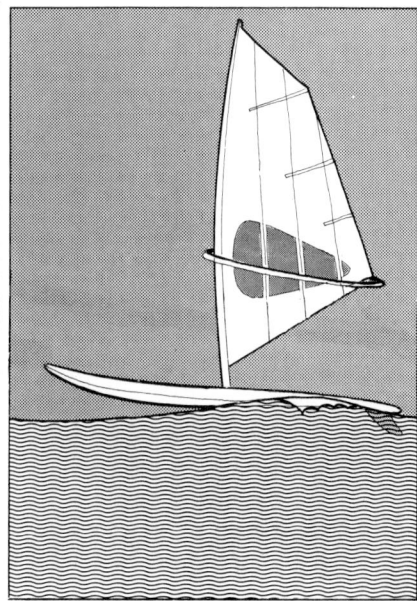

75

Seamanship

Ropes

Ropes are made of *natural fibres* (hemp and sisal) or *synthetic fibres* (polyester, polyamide or Kevlar). For surfboards, only synthetic ropes are used. Unlike natural fibres, synthetic fibres are not subject to decay and have a high resistance to fracture. Furthermore, their ends can be heat-sealed.

The fibres are either *twisted* or *woven*. For surfboards, the materials used are mostly woven and pre-stretched, as they are more flexible than twisted ropes and hold better in the cleats.

Knots and their uses

A knot must be:
● easy and quick to tie
● very stable when subjected to tension
● easy and quick to untie.

The general term "knots" includes "bends" (any knot used to fasten two ropes together) and "hitches" (a knot in which certain parts jam each other). In fact, a knot is strictly the term used for knots made in one rope. Every bend or hitch has a standing part and a running part. The standing part takes the strain and the running part is the loose end which you tie.

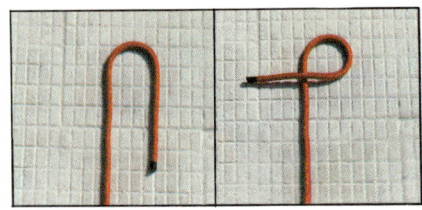

bight   eye

figure-of-eight knot

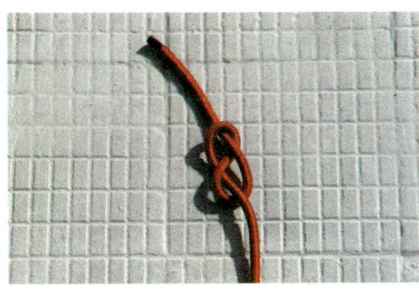

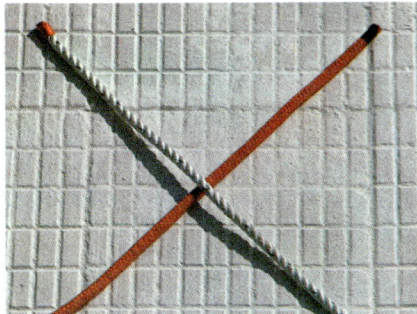

reef knot

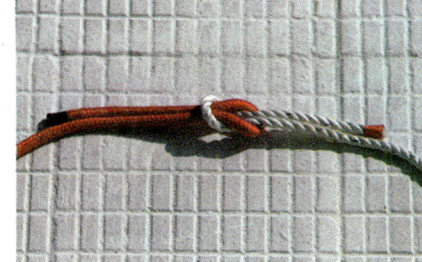

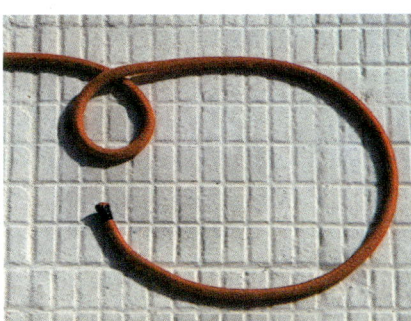

bowline

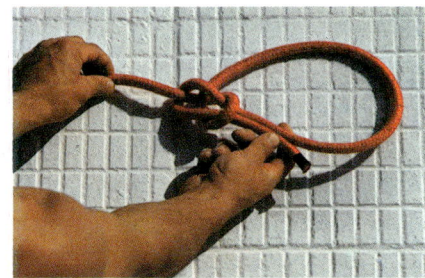

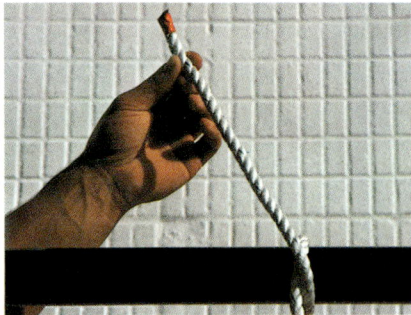

rolling hitch

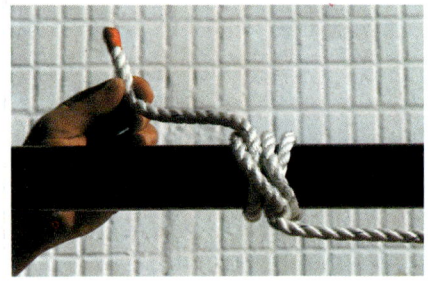

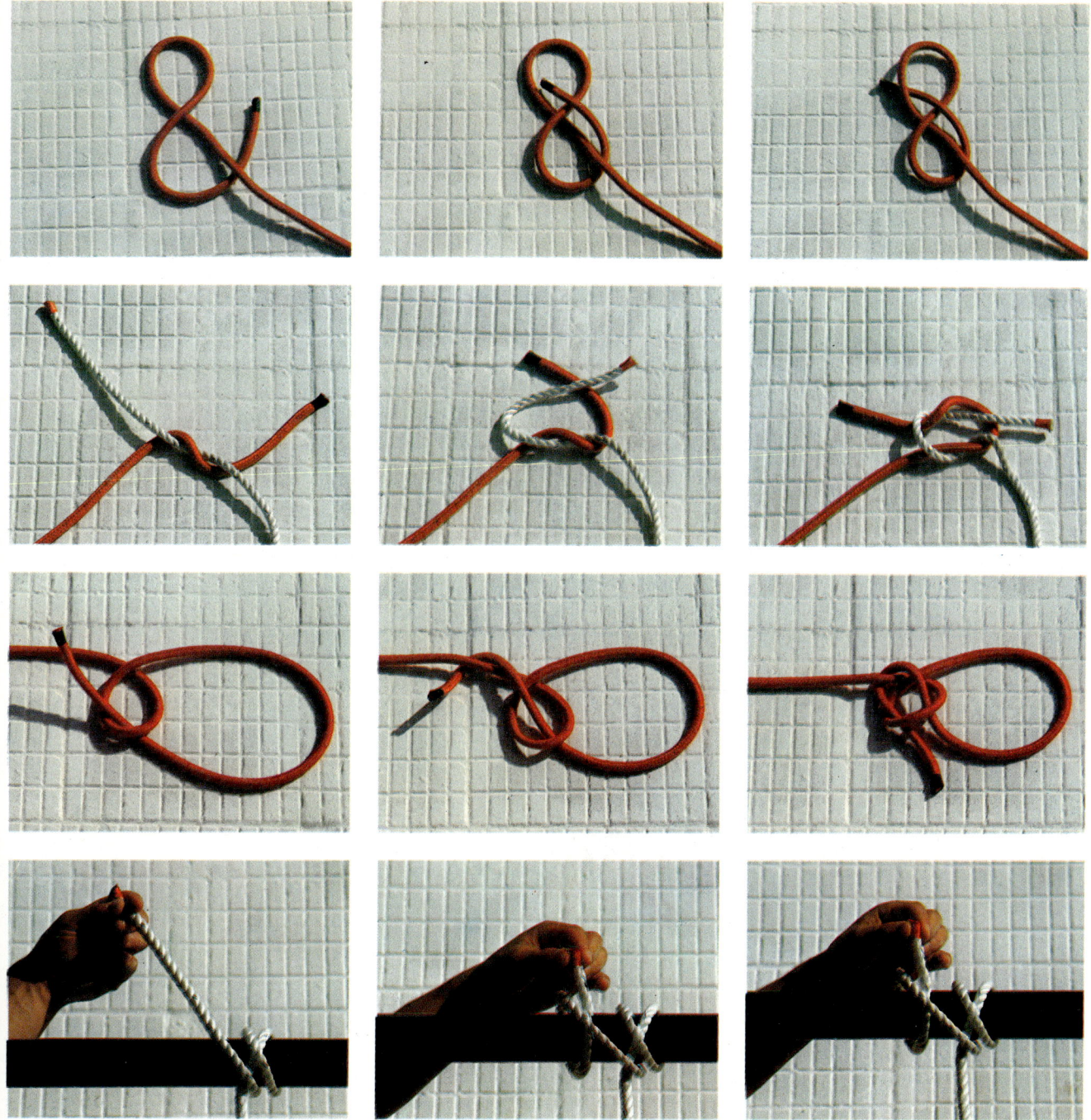

The figure-of-eight knot prevents the end from slipping out of the cleat or of another knot.

The reef knot is used to connect two ends of equal thickness.

The sheet bend. Two ends of different thickness are joined by a sheet bend.

The round turn and two half hitches can be used, among other things, for fixing the rig safety line.

The clove hitch is tied quickly and may be used to tie the folded rig together.

The rolling hitch is used to fix the mast rope to the mast.

Bowlines, or open loops, are used on the clew and on the downhaul line.

The harness knot is a figure-of-eight knot tied around the fixed end of the harness line.

Rope end protection

Every rope end must be protected against fraying. With natural fibres all rope ends have to be whipped to prevent the strands from fraying and separating. With synthetic ropes it is sufficient to heat-seal the ends together. You can do this using a candle. Make sure that the strands are pressed together tightly so that they fit in the cleats. To do this, squeeze them carefully between your wetted thumb and index finger after sealing. You can also ask your sailing and surfing specialists to trim the rope ends to the length required. The specialists use a "hot gun" with a special trimming nozzle which will ensure that the welded rope end maintains its shape.

round turn and two half hitches

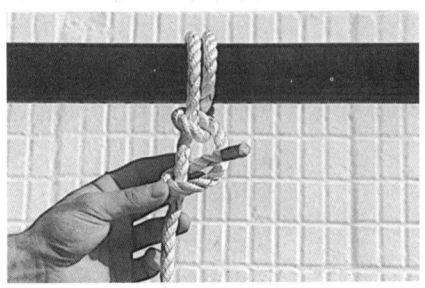
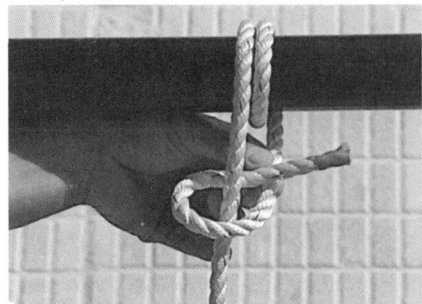

clove hitch

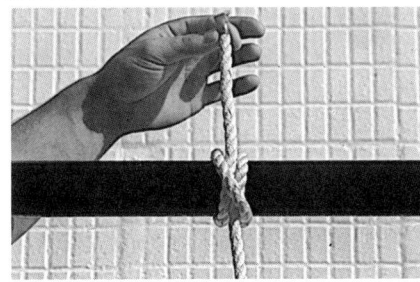
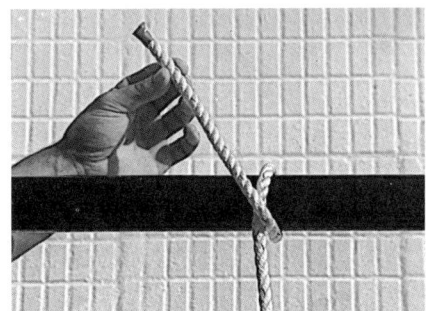

sheet bend

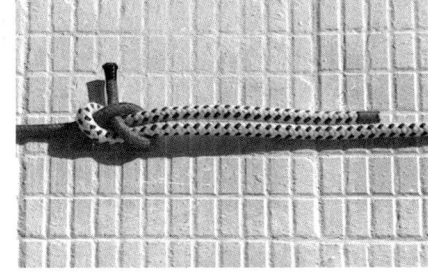
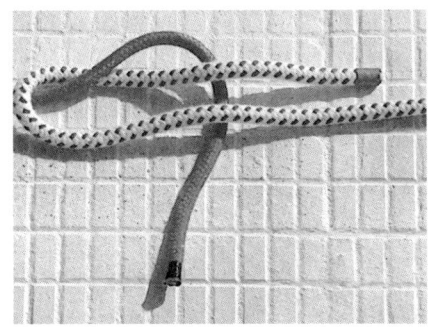

harness knot

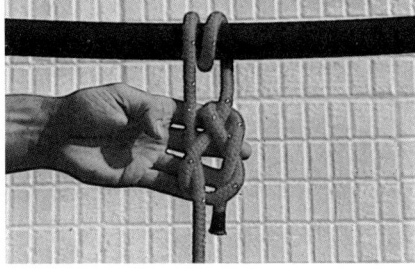
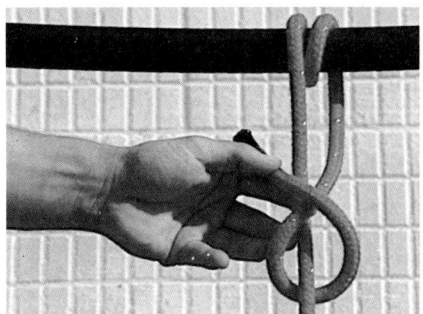

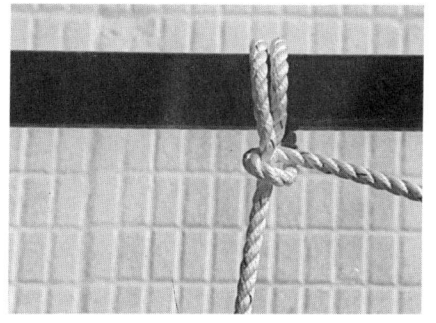

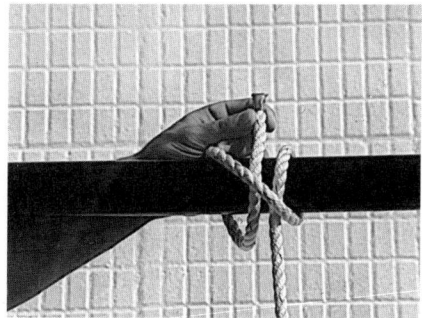

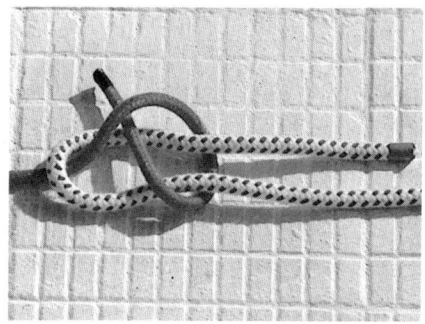

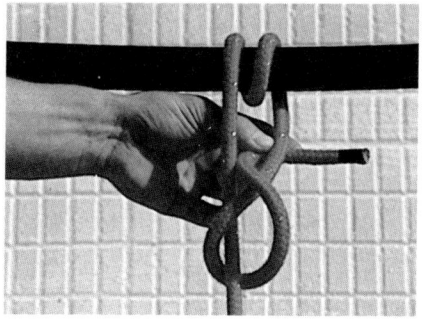

Care and repair of your surfboard

The general upkeep of a surfboard and its equipment is very simple, as it is made for the most part of synthetic materials. Thus almost all parts are service-free and you can keep your board in good condition if you observe some basic rules.

Maintenance of the board. The worst problem is when water gets into the foam. Scratches on the outer skin of the board should immediately be filled, albeit in a provisional manner (e.g. by using a filler or covering with adhesive tape). You should bear in mind that it is almost impossible to remove water from foam and that foam is destroyed by water. Also the water will expand and evaporate if the board is exposed to the sun for a long time, thus separating the foam from the skin. Even if you are not aware of having caused any damage, you should check your board regularly for hair-line cracks and wear in the gel-coat skin. It is here that water gradually seeps through, thus reducing its resilience. To prevent your board from being holed you should avoid surfing too close to the shore. Get down at the point where the water is at hip or knee depth and carry the board carefully ashore (see page 49).

On the beach you should never lay the board down on its fins and always try to keep it in the shade. Where this is impossible, lay it vertically on its side. This will prevent excessive heat on your board. Note also that materials like ABS and PE are very sensitive to ultraviolet rays. These will tend to damage toughening agents in them. In other words, frequent exposure to the sun quickly reduces their resilience.

Maintenance of the daggerboard and fin. Daggerboards and fins do not require special maintenance. If you get off your board early enough, they are protected against wear and breakage.

Wooden daggerboards should be rubbed down and given two coats of yacht varnish at regular intervals, at least at the end of the season. If there are any screws, they should be removed and the holes should be sealed with varnish.

Maintenance of the mast and the wishbone. The mast and wishbone do not require special maintenance. For your own safety, you should check them regularly for hair-line cracks or breaks. This is absolutely vital if you have fallen on the rig.

Typical points of fracture of the mast are at its lower end and at the wishbone attachment.

For the wishbone they are at the boom end fittings, the screw holes for the cleats, and the tube in the area of the harness line.

It is difficult to identify fracture marks on the mast. They are easiest to see on transparent masts, which immediately show hair-line cracks as white marks in the laminate.

When you want to check the wishbone, you should pay particular attention to the tube directly below the cleats for the outhaul line. Hang the wishbone end over a post and stretch it out a little. Cracks in the boom end fittings will open and can be recognized immediately.

On many wishbones the rubber coat becomes loose. You should glue it immediately to prevent tearing. To repair it, inject rubber adhesive underneath the rubber

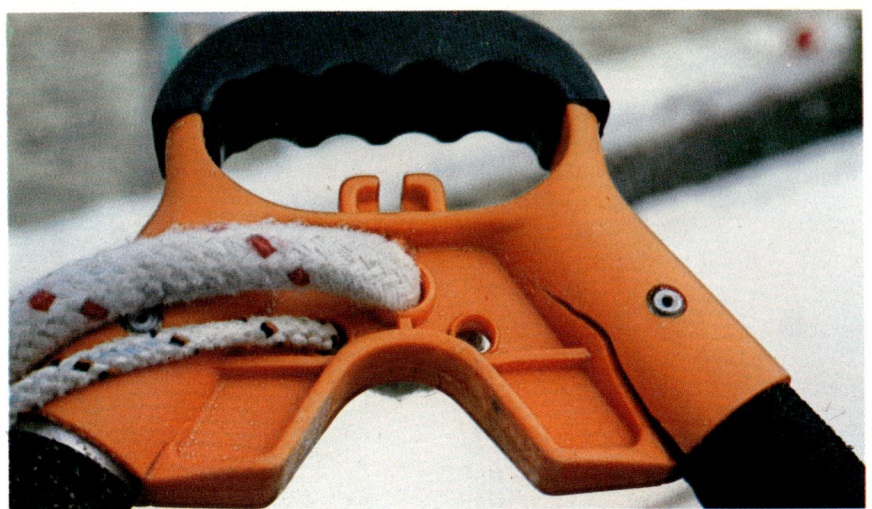

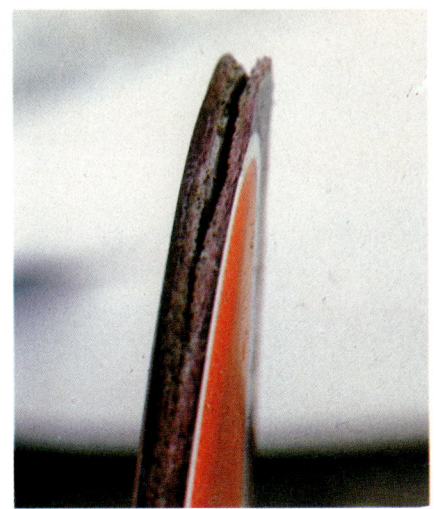

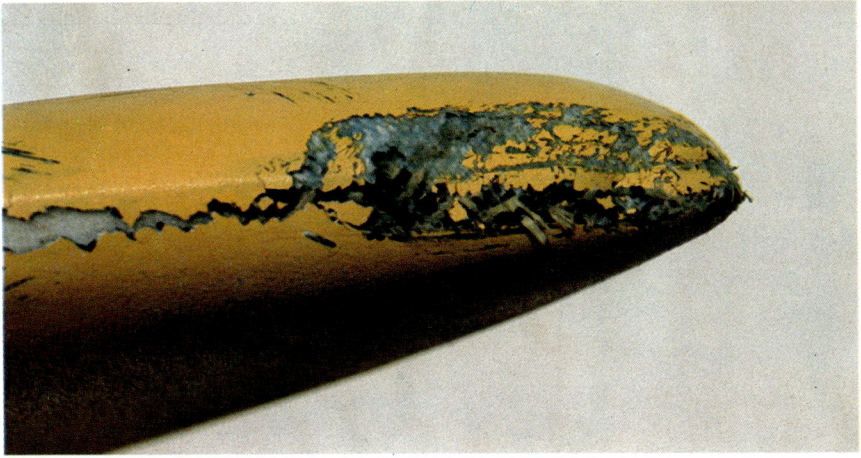

Above left: If you spread out the wishbone, the cracks in the boom end fittings will open
Above right: A fin that has hit the bottom
Left: If you leave your board too long in the water, the innards will come out

- Never leave it flapping in the wind to dry. This damages waterproofing and the stitching. Furthermore, it stretches it.
- Remove tar stains immediately. If you cannot do it straight away with dry-cleaning fluid, at least grease the tar with margarine or similar.
- When folding your sail, lay it on a clean surface – not the sand – and fold it up in "S" folds from the foot, avoiding putting a fold in the window. It is best for two people to fold it (from the foot to the head) in two or three large folds. Then fold it across (but do not bend the window; it will crack). Always fold the sail in different places or you will develop cracks there too.

(use a syringe from the chemist). Inject at four-inch intervals four times round the beam. Twist the rubber to and fro to spread the glue.

The mast foot joint requires no maintenance, but check it occasionally. If white spots appear when it is bent the rubber should be replaced. Check rivets and screws for proper fitting.

Surfing suits must be protected from strong sunlight and always rinsed in fresh water after use. Laminated suits should be rubbed with talcum powder and zips greased occasionally.

Care of the sail This is the most fragile piece of your equipment and the one most likely to be damaged. Follow this drill after you have used it:

- Wash it as soon as possible in lots of fresh water. Salt burns pinholes in it even when dry.

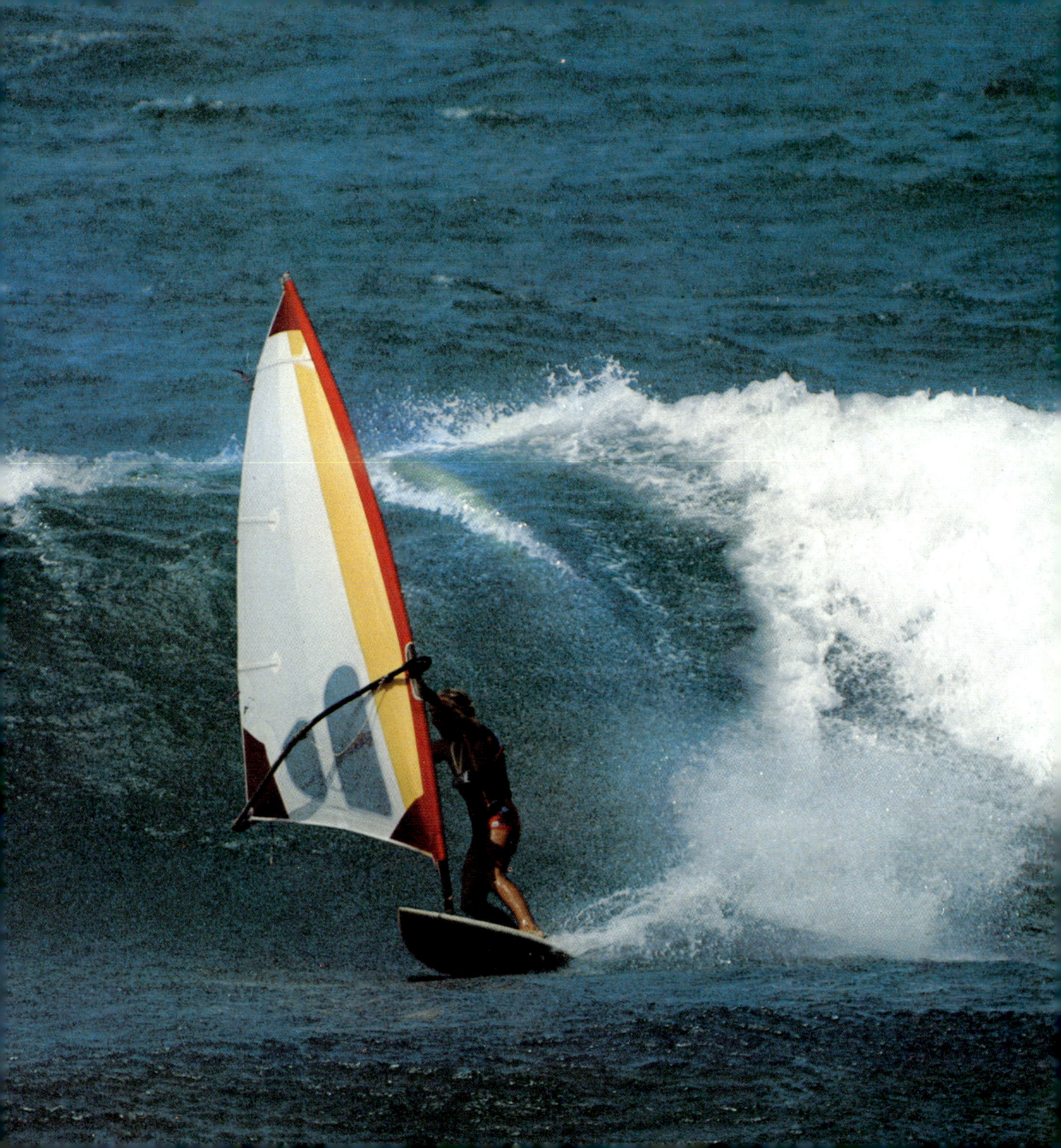

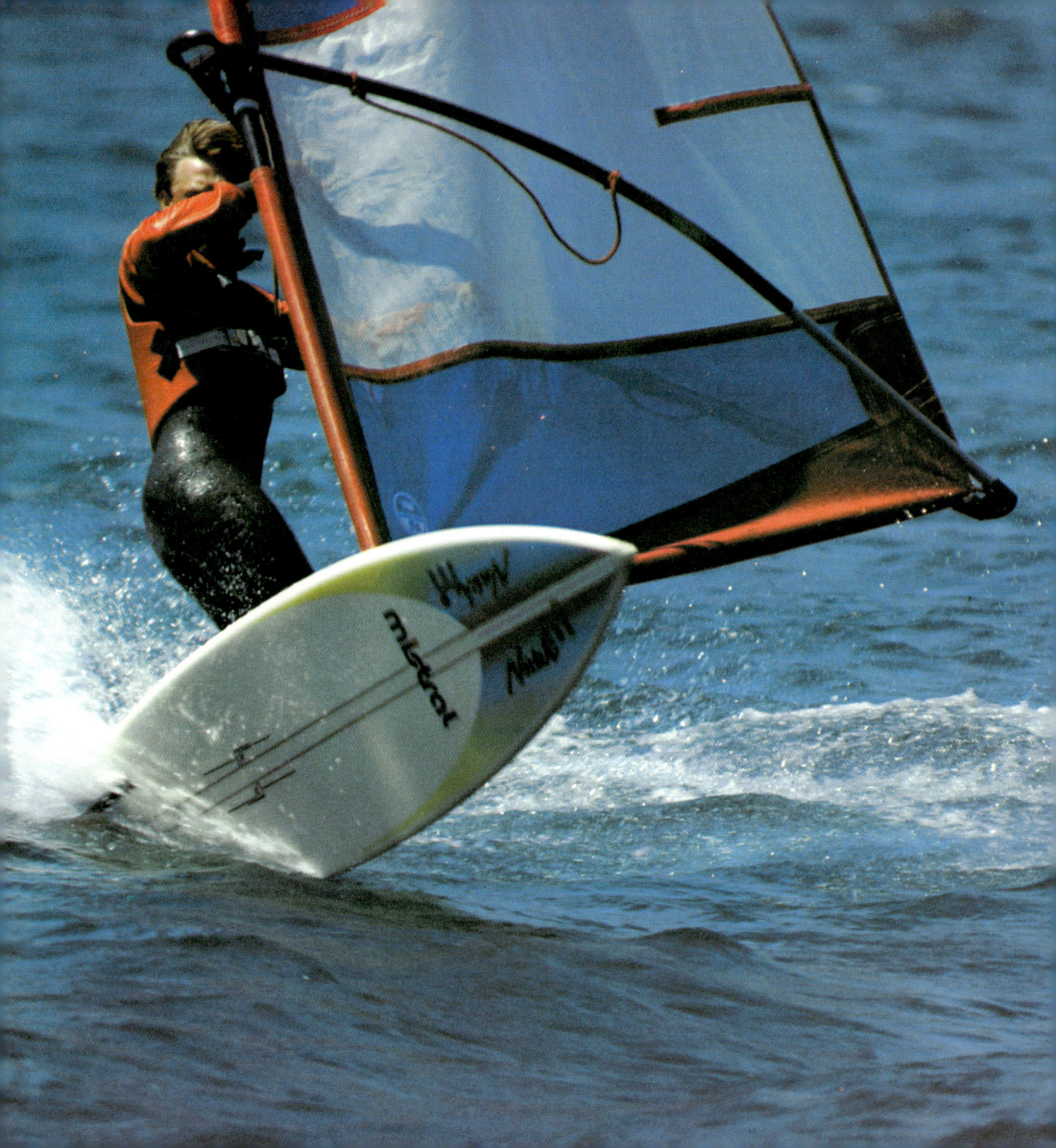

Rules and regulations

Just as on the road, there are rules about collision which you must obey. A sailboard has been known to sink a yacht!

International Collision Regulations

There are 38 "Rules of the road" on the water. So far as you are concerned it is very unlikely that you will sail in shipping channels far out at sea but in harbours and estuaries you *will* meet the largish stuff. The captains, be they amateur or professional, will expect you to obey the rules. Although "power gives way to sail" in open waters, the reverse is true in restricted channels. No big yacht is going to run aground to avoid you. So the best advice is to keep out of shipping channels which are marked with green and red buoys close to

harbours. Coming in from the sea, the ships will see green buoys on the right of their channel and red ones on the left.

These rules even operate on Lake Windemere and other large waters in the United Kingdom. On rivers there are usually special rules in addition but generally everybody keeps to the right-hand side of the river or canal and you can expect them to do so. So you hastily keep clear.

Well! What do you do when you meet another sailboard or sailing vessel of any kind?

There are three rules which you *must* know:

● When two *sailing* vessels meet, and each has the wind on a different side, the vessel which has the wind on the port side shall keep out of the way of the other. So a sailing vessel, including a sailboard, which is on starboard tack, has priority and the others must keep out of the way. This is invariably the rule, except when the larger vessel may run aground if it is forced out of a narrow channel.

● The second rule as between *sailing* vessels is that when both have the wind on the same side, the vessel which is to windward shall keep out of the way of the vessel that is to leeward. All you have to do when sailing along parallel to another board is to decide that *he* is nearer to the wind – it will get to him first. Then *he* must keep out of *your* way. Of course, the reverse may be true! If necessary, the give-way vessel may have to tack or turn around to go right under the stern of the other.

● The third important rule which applies both to power and sailing

vessels is: an overtaking vessel shall keep clear. This is the most obvious since you do not have eyes in the back of your head.

Whatever the actual rules say, there is also a general rule which says that it is the duty of every mariner to avoid collision. The other man may not have seen you – quite possible in a larger vessel – so don't rely on him to avoid collision. You have a duty too. So if you are going to change course (and it is easy for you to do so quickly on a sailboard) do it firmly, boldly and in ample time to clear. Remember that the wind may suddenly die away and there you will be, bobbing helplessly in the path of a large vessel which may be expecting you to "do the correct thing".

Road rules

There are some points to remember other than the normal Highway Code, when you are roof-racking your board.

● Strong rack, properly clamped on.
● Board tightly strapped and padded.
● Board inverted, facing at the front to help prevent it lifting at speed.
● Line from bow to front bumper.
● Boom on top or underneath board.
● Mast in special mast fitting, or, if none, then *securely* fastened – without the sail on it. It is bad for the sail.
● If your front or rear projection is greater than 1.07 m (3′ 6″) it must be marked with a red marker clearly visible at night.
● The law is very general, and you can be prosecuted for "an unsafe load".

Important "water rules"

Between sailing vessels
● Starboard tack has priority
● Windward board keeps clear
● Overtaking board keeps clear

Between boards and other vessels
● Do not impede the passage of a vessel which can safely navigate only within a narrow channel or fairway.
● Do not cross in front of, or sail too close to, a vessel larger than a board.
● Change course firmly, boldly and in ample time to make your intentions clear.
● Watch out for swimmers when sailing your board.

Philip Pudenz gybing

83

Racing

A windsurfing regatta consists of several races. In most international regattas, there are seven, of which six count. In championships, at least five races are required, of which four count.

A race starts, unless otherwise announced, five minutes before the start signal and ends when the finish line is crossed. To ascertain the overall winner from the places in the individual races, places are allocated points. The International Yacht Racing Union lays down the international regulations for racing and each national authority adds certain clauses to suit local conditions. Clubs running races will issue sailing instructions for each race.

The course

Usually the course to be sailed is the *Olympic triangle*, which consists of the start directly into the wind, the broad reach to the reaching mark, the opposite reach to the bottom mark, the second beat up to the top mark, the running and the final beat up to the finish. In smaller races, contestants often sail a further triangle.

The start and finish lines

The start and finish lines are marked by two buoys in a line or alternatively by a buoy and the start/finish vessel. In all other cases, the start line is marked by the leeward buoy (bottom mark) and the start vessel. The finish line is marked by the windward buoy (top mark) and the finish vessel.

The starting procedure with fixed starting line

In windsurfing and yachting regattas, flying starts are used, i.e. the competitors try to cross the start line at optimum speed when the starting gun is fired.

Ten minutes before the start, the *preliminary signal* is given, i.e. a gun is fired and the course-indicating and class flags are hoisted. Five minutes before the start the *preparatory signal* is given, i.e. a gun is fired and the Blue Peter is hoisted. The race has now started and the race regulations apply.

The *start signal* itself is a gun, with simultaneous lowering of all flags which had been hoisted.

Premature starts

Sailors who start prematurely are recalled for an orderly start by flying the flag X. They have no right of way until they have crossed the start line properly. If several boats start prematurely and they cannot be identified, the signal *"General recall"* is given. In most cases the *One Minute Rule* applies, i. e. boards which cross the line in the last minute before the start are disqualified unless they round the outside of the starting line and return to the starting area.

Definitions

When racing, it is important to know exactly when a board has been overtaken by another. A board is *clear astern* of another if its bow has not crossed an imaginary line at right angles to the other's stern. When that happens, his duty to keep clear ends and other rules begin to apply. If three boards are together the last is "connected" to the first by the intermediate one and an

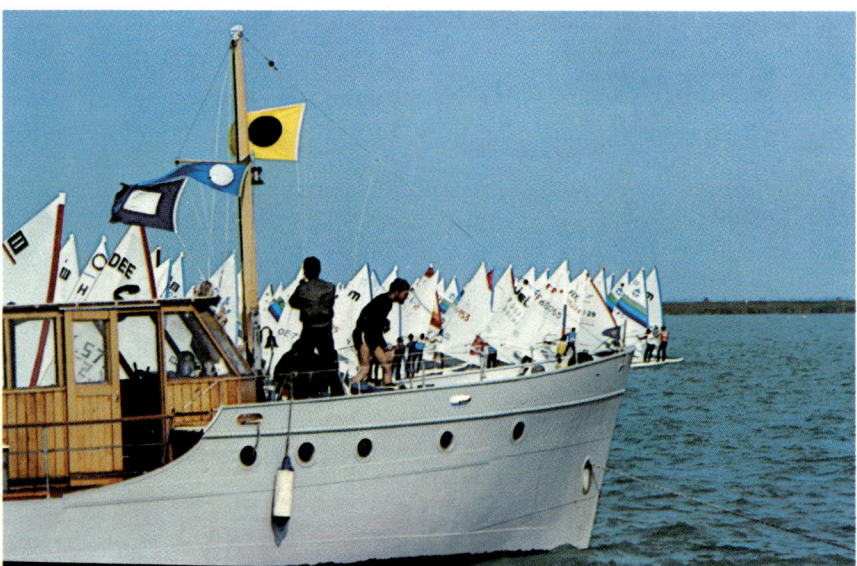

The start of a regatta in the Open Class. The flags are already being hauled down on the start vessel. On the left, you can see the Blue Peter and on the right Flag 1 (One minute Rule)

overlap can occur between first and last. Rather complicated, but all explained in the Racing Rules and, if you are going to race, you can get simplified rules from the Royal Yachting Association. Another definition of importance is *correct course* – that is, the course a board would take to sail a race as fast as possible.

Rules for giving way

The rules for giving way are almost exactly the same as we have discussed earlier. A boat on starboard tack has priority over one on the port tack. A windward boat must keep clear of one that is to leeward.

The boat with right of way must maintain its course, or if it does not, then it must give warning.

Only the rule for overtaking is slightly different because, when competing, it is good tactics to overtake to windward and take the wind out of the other board's sail. The board which is overtaken may retaliate by beating to windward, at will and without warning. This is called a *luffing match*. It comes to an end when the overtaking boat succeeds in reaching the *mast abeam position*. This position is reached when the overtaking sailor is level with the mast of the craft overtaken. He then shouts "mast abeam" and the overtaken craft must fall off to its correct course.

Rounding a mark. If a buoy is touched or rounded wrongly, it must be rounded a second time.

If several boards intend to round a mark simultaneously, the rule that the craft on starboard tack has right of way over the craft on port tack applies to boards which have the wind blowing from different sides. If the sails are luffed on the same side, then the inner board has right of way provided that it could overlap the other board two board lengths before the mark.

Keeping clear during manoeuvres. When you are tacking or gybing, you must keep clear of other contestants. A tack starts when the board is at a right angle to the wind and is finished

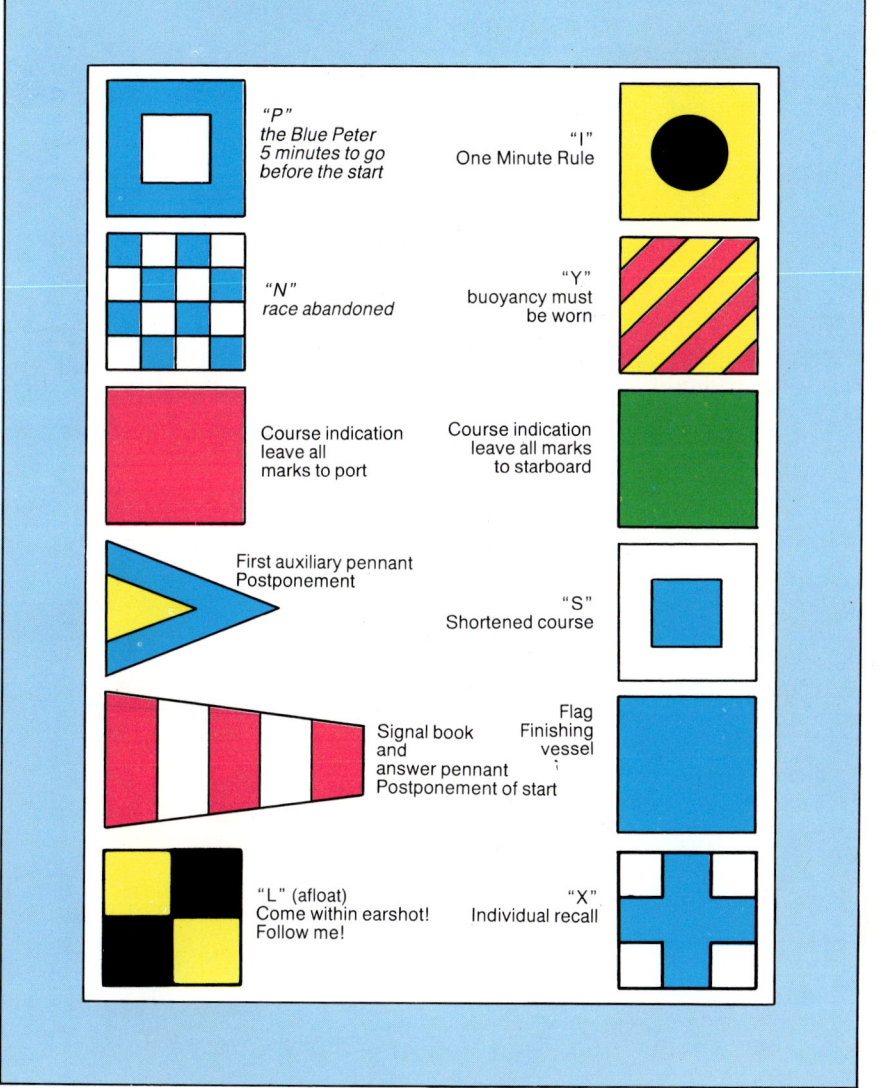

"P" the Blue Peter 5 minutes to go before the start

"I" One Minute Rule

"N" race abandoned

"Y" buoyancy must be worn

Course indication leave all marks to port

Course indication leave all marks to starboard

First auxiliary pennant Postponement

"S" Shortened course

Signal book and answer pennant Postponement of start

Flag Finishing vessel

"L" (afloat) Come within earshot! Follow me!

"X" Individual recall

The most important flags and pennants used in regattas

when the sail is full again. A gybe lasts from the time when the wishbone crosses the midship line until the sail is full again on the new tack.

You are not allowed to demand space immediately after a manoeuvre.

The "720". If you have caused a collision you can absolve yourself by executing a *720-degree turn* at the next reasonable opportunity. When turning, you must keep clear of other contestants.

Protests must be handed in to the regatta organisers in writing and a protest fee must be deposited. Which statements must be given can be seen in the protest forms.

Behaviour of other sportsmen on the water towards regatta sailors. Regatta contestants are obliged to observe the Rules of the Road when meeting swimmers or other craft not participating in the regatta.

Certificates of competence

Unlike many other countries, the United Kingdom has no compulsory certificates of competence but this does not mean that the Government has not bothered to take care of its citizens.

When windsurfing or boardsailing started in the United Kingdom the RYA took up the already established scheme run by the International Windsurfer Schools and there are now many, many recognised schools where people can learn.

Progress in the Scheme
The structure of the Royal Yachting

Association scheme is simple. For the beginner, the National Boardsailing Award provides a good background of practical experience.

The next step is the optional "Improvers" Course and finally the "Advanced Open Sea Award" or the "Advanced Inland Award" may be achieved.

What is particularly attactive about the scheme is that, on completion, the Personal Logbook which you will have kept may be useful if you want to advance to Instructor status and perhaps even more useful if you take your board abroad.

Small Craft Register
Although nobody demands that you register your sailboard as a Small Ship it is perfectly possible to do so. But frankly, at present, not very necessary because most Customs officials and others in authority consider that a sailboard is hardly more important to check on than the contents of your suitcase.

The classes of surfboard
In order to be able to organise windsurfing events in which the technical proficiency of the competitors is assessed, the boards must be compatible with each other. For this purpose, the associations who organise competitions determine classes of windsurfing boards according to their specific properties.

One design. Boards which belong to this class are manufactured according to uniform construction plans. The sizes of the rig and board, the weight, and even such details as permission to use rubber lines as a connection to the uphaul rope are all laid down. The Windsurfer is an example.

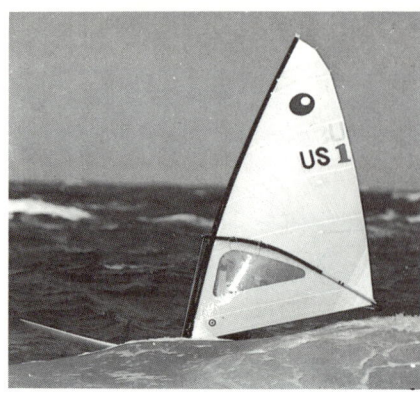

Ken Winner's sail displays the Bic Marine logo, the nationality (USA) and his sailing number.

IWGCA
International Windglider Class Association
Rottink Travel Agency Building
Prinses Irenestraat 31
1077 WV Amsterdam
Netherlands.

IWCA
International Windsurfer Class Association
1955 West 190th St
Torrance CA 90509
USA

IMCO
International Mistral Class Association
Herengracht 52P
1015 BN Amsterdam
Netherlands

IBSA
International Boardsailing Association
PO Box 1710
CH-3001 Bern
Switzerland

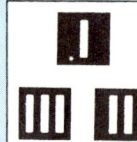

The construction class defines the limits which must not be exceeded. Within these, there are no restrictions on constructional inventiveness.

Single type classes. Following the formation of a class association, various requirements have to be met (e.g. a minimum of 100 members) and tests on the regulations concerning classes and measurements have to be passed.

National classes. The single type class is the preliminary stage before a class is accepted as a national class.

International classes must be in existence in several countries and represented by a class organisation. They are recognised by the International Yacht Racing Union.

The Olympic classes. After the Olympic Games the sailing boats classes for the next games are chosen.

The recognised classes of windsurfing boards. You will find the recognised classes of windsurfing boards in the table on the left, together with their class marks.

Every board type and class has sail insignia. **Sail insignia** consist of a *class mark* (see left for illustrations), the *sailing number* (in most cases this is the number allocated by the board manufacturer or the number registered with the regional association) and the *nationality mark* (e.g. a G for the Federal Republic of Germany, K for Great Britain etc.)

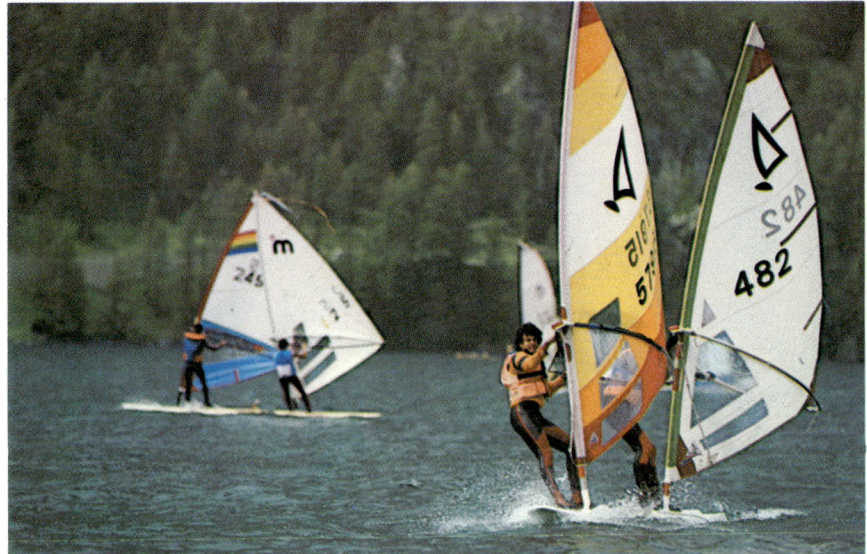

Other forms of sailboarding

Tandem surfing
Team-work between the two partners makes this sport one of the most sociable forms.

Freestyle
A freestyle surfer turns his board into a platform on which he performs

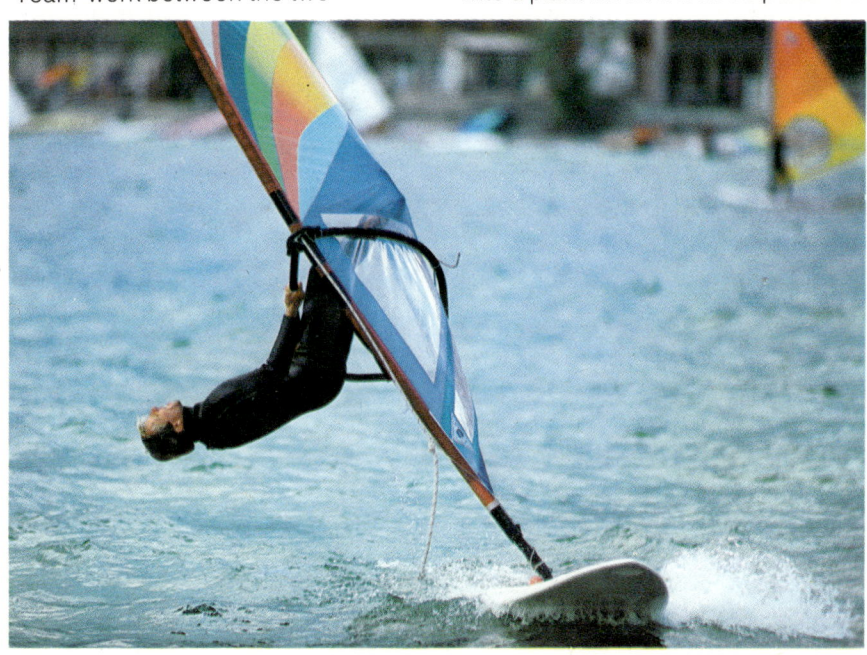

87

tricks. Water starts, rail-riding and sailing with your body inside the wishbone are less difficult tricks, but upward circles and somersaults are only for real experts.

years, they have become the ultimate in sail boards.

Wave sailing

Wave sailing is every windsurfer's

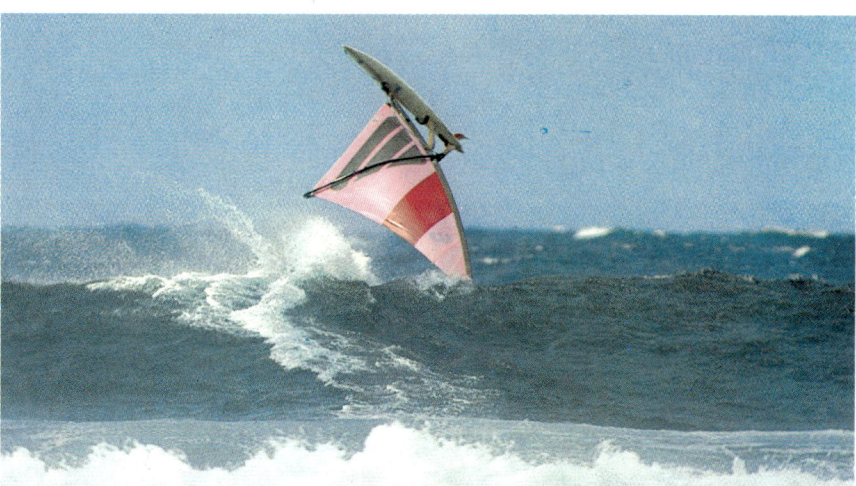

Funboard surfing

Funboard surfing brings the sport full circle back to its origins: namely surfriding. The dimensions of funboards have become increasingly similar to those of surfriding boards. In the last few

dream. Hawaii has become a kind of Promised Land. But be careful. Do not let these pictures tempt you. The waters of Sunset Beach or the Hookipa waves make severe demands on even world-class surfers, and even they have to take

their courage in both hands. You should rather choose smaller waves appropriate to your knowledge and skill. Otherwise you risk your equipment, your safety and your life.

Surfing on ice

When winter comes, the surfing season is far from being finished. Some move to warmer regions, others take to the ice. Surfing on ice is the fastest way of moving in an upright position using a sail. Speed is much faster than that of the wind. In a force 4 breeze, speeds of 40 to 50 mph can be achieved. Therefore you should take precautions against

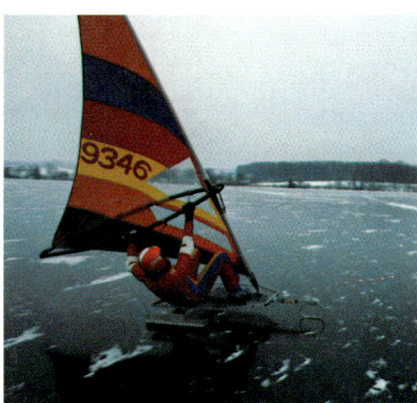

a possible fall. Your knees and elbows must be well protected, and you should wear a helmet. It goes without saying, that gloves and warm clothing are necessary. Otherwise your injuries will be more than just bruises.

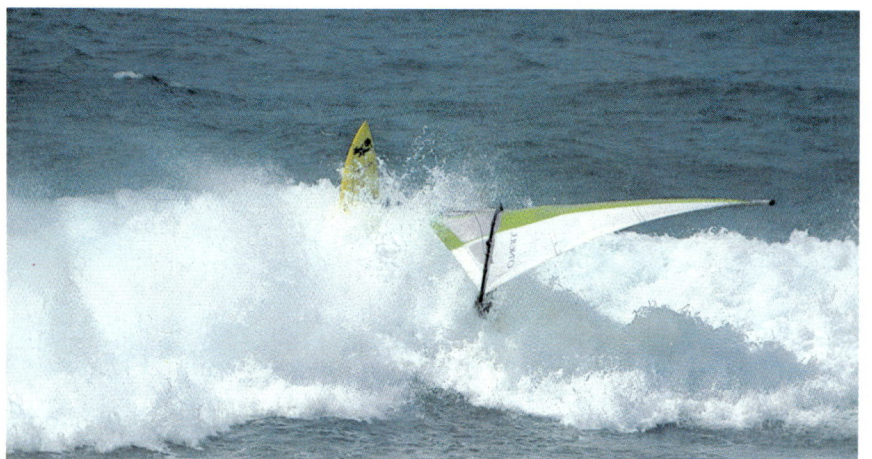

Windsurfing and the environment

In recent years damage to the environment and its various causes have been the subject of frequent discussions.

You may be surprised to read that of late the windsurfer has come under attack as the cause of harm to the environment. It remains to be seen whether or not this is justified. In any case you as a windsurfer should be aware of your share in our responsibility for preserving nature. You can take your board sailing anywhere, which means that you can go windsurfing almost anywhere, even in places where nobody has ever been sailing before and which were reserved to wild fowl and fish as breeding and spawning areas. Through carelessness you may very quickly cause irreparable damage to hitherto intact ecosystems. So you should read the following rules very carefully and observe them when practising your sport.

10 Golden Rules to safeguard the environment*

1. Be careful not to sail into reeds and overgrown sections on the water's edge. Avoid pebble, mud and sand banks, i.e. places where birds feed and make their nests. Avoid shallow waters, i.e. spawning areas, and in particular areas with water plants.
2. Keep a sufficient distance from reeds and overgrown sections on the water's edge, e.g. 30 to 50 m on large rivers. Keep a sufficient distance from flocks of birds on the water, if possible more than 100 m.
3. Strictly observe regulations in force in nature conservation areas. It is frequently the case in conservation areas that water sports are prohibited throughout the year, or at least during special seasons; if they are not prohibited completely, it may be they are only permitted under certain conditions. White-water canoeists must not alter the river bed, e.g. by removing obstructing rocks.
4. Be particularly careful in "wetlands of international importance". These areas are the biosphere of rare animals and plants and require protection.
5. Go ashore only in places which are marked as landing places or where it is clear that no damage can be done.
6. When you are ashore, do not go near reeds and other overgrown sections on the water's edge, in order not to invade and threaten the habitats of birds, fish, microbiota and plants.
7. Do not sail near areas in intertidal zones where seals live, in order not to disturb or drive them away. Keep a distance of at least 300 to 500 yards from seal and bird resting areas. Never leave the marked channel. Sail slowly.
8. Watch and take photos of animals only from a distance.
9. Keep the water clean. Waste, e.g. the contents of chemical toilets, must never be dumped in the water. This waste must be disposed of at special collection points in ports in the same way as used oils are. In ports, only use the sanitary facilities on land. When laid up, do not keep the motor running, to avoid environmental damage through waste gases.
10. When these rules apply to you, observe them. Make sure you know all the applicable regulations for your particular sport. See to it that your knowledge and your exemplary behaviour and attitude towards nature is passed on to young people and less enlightened water sportsmen.

* Most of these rules have been taken up by governments, and are now law. In many cases there are penalties for infringement.

Tides

tide	ebb and flood
flood	rising water
ebb	receding water
high tide/water	the time of highest water level (between two tides)
low tide/water	the time of lowest water level
tidal range	the difference in height between high and low waters
spring tide	particularly high tidal range (lasts 4 days)
mid-extreme tide	three days between spring tide and neap tides with normal range
neap tide	particularly low tidal range (lasts 4 days)

Two phenomena resulting from the tides, namely the changing water level and the resulting currents, may either be of very great benefit to the windsurfer or a source of considerable danger.

Tides are the result of the gravitational forces between the moon and the earth. The sun exerts additional influence. On that area of the earth above which the moon is orbiting at any given time, the water heaps up, which is called flood tide. As a kind of compensation water will also heap up on the opposite side of the earth. Every 25 hours, the earth has completed a full circle under the moon, so that flood tides occur every 12 ½ hours. Despite the fact that water particles move along with the rotation of the earth — they hardly change their position relative to the earth — high waters will always heap up in the direction of the gravitational attraction of the moon. Since we move together with the rotation of the earth, we get the impression that the water

The earth moves under the gravitational attraction of the moon and thus underneath the flood

approaches during flood tides and recedes during ebb tides. In reality, however, high waters heap up and remain stationary under the influence of the moon.

An example may clarify this: when water slops to and fro in a bucket, not one water particle will move from the left edge to the right, although you might say one side has a "low tide" and the other a "high tide". The particles move only as much as necessary to raise the level slightly on one side, and to lower it on the other side. If we compare the surface of the oceans with the surface of the water in the bucket, the tides would change the level near the edges of the bucket by less than one thousandth millionth of a millimetre. This corresponds to an average of 5 metres of changing water levels on the earth.

Spring tides and neap tides

Spring tides and neap tides are caused by the influence of the sun.

The position of earth, sun and moon affects the phases of the moon and the spring tide

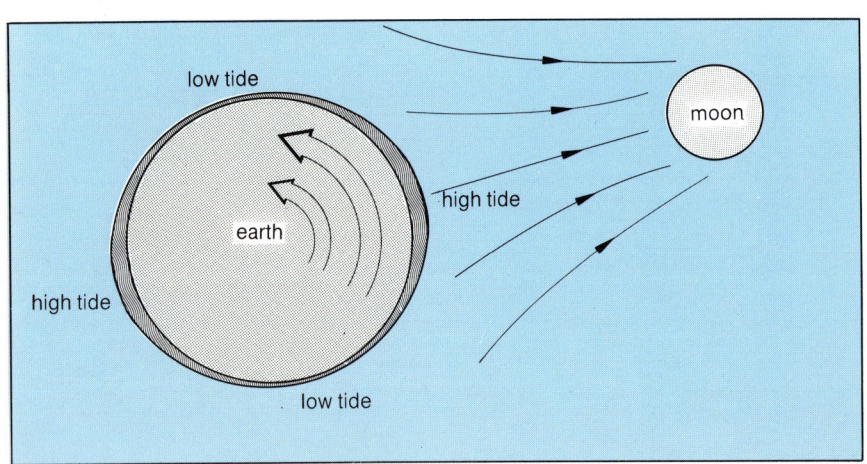

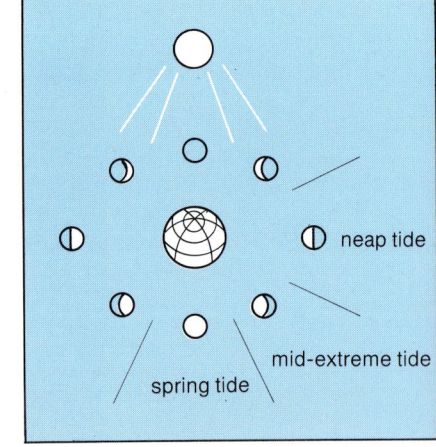

When the sun forms an axis with the moon and the earth, it adds to the influence of the moon. Spring tides occur. High tides are higher and low tides lower than normal. This is called an extreme tidal range. When the sun is perpendicular to the earth-moon axis, high tides are extremely low and low tides are extremely high. This is the neap tide and the tidal range is small. The tide between spring and neap tides is called the mid-extreme tide, during which the sun has no influence.

As the constellation cycle of sun, moon and earth recurs every two weeks, the change in the tides can be calculated in advance. Four days of spring tide are followed by three days of mid-extreme tide, after which come four days of neap tide, and again three days of mid-extreme tide.

As can be seen in the illustration, at full moon and new moon spring tides should occur and at half moon, neap tides. However, continents impede the tidal currents, so that on Europe's coasts, tides are delayed against the phases of the moon. The tidal epoch for most of the North Sea coast, for example, is recorded as being two days, which means that the tide only reaches its highest point two days after full moon.

The Tide Tables

Tide Tables are published in many forms in the United Kingdom, but can be found in Nautical Almanacs for yachtsmen. Dover is used as one standard port and many other principal ports are shown in full. The almanacs also contain tables of tidal constants for a large number of smaller ports for which the full tide tables are not published. Suppose we wish to find the time of High Water at a little port near Dover called Hole Haven. If we look it up we will find that its constant is shown as + 1 hour 23 minutes. Read the Dover tables and add 1 hour 23 minutes to the Dover figures. If you are sailing in only one area quite regularly you will be able

An example of a tide table for September				
Day	September			
	High Water		Low Water	
	time	time	time	time
1 W	11.36		5.59	18.29
2 T	0.07	12.18	6.43	19.08
3 F2	0.44	12.56	7.22	19.46
4 S	1.19	13.32	7.59	20.23
5 S	1.55	14.06	8.34	20.57
6 M	2.29	14.40	9.06	21.30
7 T	3.04	15.15	9.39	22.05
8 W	3.40	15.53	10.16	22.42
9 T	4.18	16.33	10.55	23.19
10 F3	4.56	17.14	11.33	23.56
11 S	5.37	18.06		12.20
12 S	6.35	19.20	0.48	13.30
13 M	7.56	20.53	2.07	15.02
14 T	9.28	22.21	3.43	16.37
15 W	10.48	23.30	5.09	17.52
16 T	11.49		6.14	18.48
17 F0	0.24	12.38	7.05	19.36
18 S	1.09	13.21	7.51	20.20
19 S	1.50	14.03	8.34	21.00
20 M	2.30	14.42	9.12	21.35
21 T	3.07	15.19	9.46	22.07
22 W	3.41	15.53	10.17	22.27
23 T	4.12	16.27	10.47	23.04
24 F	4.43	17.02	11.18	23.32
25 S1	5.18	17.45	11.55	
26 S	5.06	17.45	0.12	11.50
27 M	6.16	19.07	0.16	13.09
28 T	7.42	20.35	1.45	14.42
29 W	9.03	21.48	3.15	16.01
30 T	10.03	22.38	4.25	16.57

0: New moon
1: 1st Quarter
2: Full moon
3: Last Quarter

Central European Summer Time up to 3am on 26th September, thereafter Central European Winter Time

Tide Differences		
Place	High Water	Low Water
	h min	h min
Lister Basin		
Fairway Buoy	+ 1 47	
List West	+ 1 56	+ 1 36
List	+ 2 46	+ 2 08
Munkmarsch	+ 2 50	+ 2 10
Hindenburgdamm −Nord	+ 2 55	
Westerland	+ 0 53	+ 1 13
Vortrapp Basin		
Amrum		
Knispsand	+ 1 35	+ 1 25
Odde	+ 1 58	
Hörnum Basin		
Hörnum Odde	+ 1 54	+ 1 19
Hörnum Harbour	+ 2 19	+ 1 39

to obtain the local tide tables on a card from the local chandlery or the Harbour Master's office.

Tidal currents

Off-shore islands, shallow off-shore waters, and estuaries impede tidal currents and divert them from their normal channel. This results in strong and often unpredictable currents. In the Channel, tidal ranges can reach 10 m, whereas they are only 3 m high in the German Bight. But despite this, it is possible to observe a regular cycle of tides.

The illustration shows that during high tide and low tide the hourly rate of change in the water level is only slight. However, between high and low tides the level changes three times as quickly in an hour, and with it the force of the current.

Between Sylt and Römö, for example, currents run at 8 km/h (5 mph). For you as a surfer this means that in a quarter of an hour you will drift off over a mile and will no longer be visible from the shore.

The direction of the current does not always correspond to the direction of the tide. When the bottom of the sea or shore formations obstruct the water from flowing away, the water may flow towards the shore at low tide and seaward at high tide respectively.

Never forget to ask local people about such matters. They can give you vital information in many cases.

Special currents may occur in tidelands. During low tide, tideways collect all the water of the tideland. Larger tideways are marked for shipping with buoys and perches, but on long exposed beaches you may often find unusual and rapid cross currents which can be very

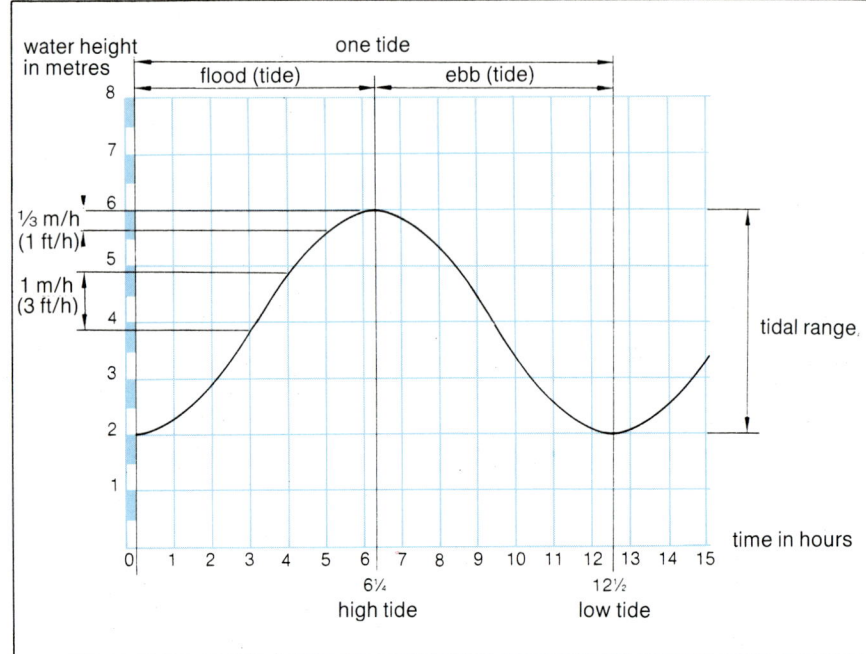

dangerous. You can ask fishermen, or at any rate local windsurfing schools, for details about the peculiarities of the currents in that area.

The steepest part of the graph shows the biggest changes in water level and hence the strongest currents

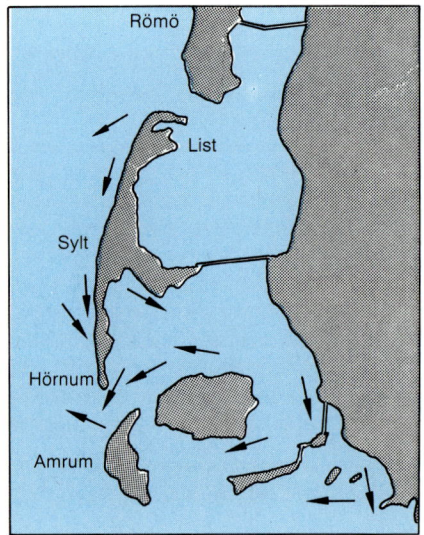

The weather

Windsurfing is dependent in the first instance on the weather and hence the wind. Weather forecasts make it easier for you to plan your windsurfing outing and make surfing tours safe. This is easier said than done, you may think, when forecasters are often incapable of making accurate forecasts.

For large areas, it is difficult to assess the air movements continuously circulating in the earth's atmosphere, and producing wind and weather. For small areas,

Currents in the area of Sylt at ebb tide, 4 hours after high tide

these movements are easy to understand.

Important factors in predicting how the weather will develop are the pressure, the temperature and the humidity of the air. From these the meteorologist will calculate the general weather situation at the time. When in addition to that, you watch wind and cloud development, you can get a more accurate picture, with which you can make correct forecasts for your own locality.

The general weather situation

The weather chart depicts the weather at a given moment, from which possible developments can be deduced. The energy brought by the sun's rays creates areas of cold and warm air. The warm air rises and leaves a relative vacuum behind. In other areas, the cold air subsides to form an area of high pressure. This is how a low (pressure area) and a high (pressure area) come into existence.

The atmospheric (barometric) pressure is measured in and around these areas, and all places showing equal pressure are connected by isobar lines on the weather chart.

These lines are entered on the weather chart at intervals of 5 mbar, so that they enclose the centres of the pressure areas, forming irregular circles.

The pressure differences in a high and a low tend to even each other out. The air flows from the high pressure area to the low pressure area. If the isobars are closer together the pressure gradient is higher and the resulting air current, i.e. the wind, is stronger. A distance between isobars of 200 km (from the North Sea coast to Hanover) means an enormous pressure gradient, and winds of up to Force 8

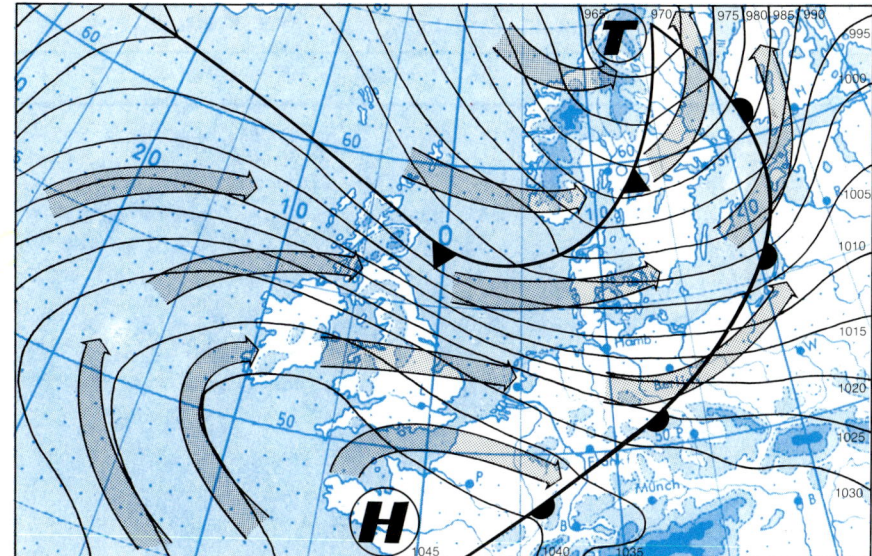

on the Beaufort Scale are to be expected. A distance of 400 km means Force 4 to 5, and one of 600 km means Force 2.

Influenced by the rotation of the earth, the air currents are deflected from their direct path towards the low and thus flow in spirals to the centre of the low (anti-clockwise in the northern hemisphere). The currents also flow in a spiral out of the high (clockwise in the northern hemisphere).

The deflection is so strong that the wind near the surface of the earth blows at an angle of 10 to 20 degrees, i.e. nearly parallel to the isobars.

The weather charts issued by weather centres will provide exact information on the atmospheric pressure and temperature, and special symbols indicating cloud cover and the speed and direction of the wind.

Weather Chart issued by German Weather Service on 21.1.1983

Key to symbols

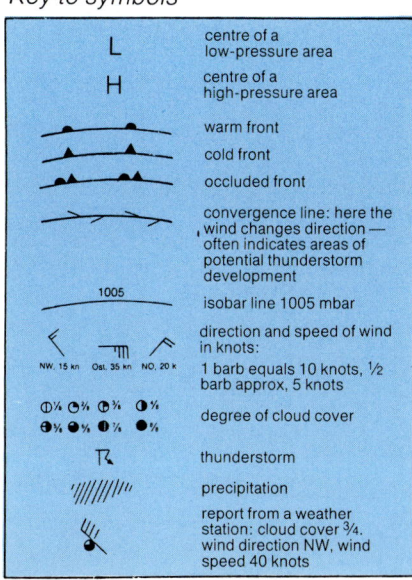

L	centre of a low-pressure area
H	centre of a high-pressure area
	warm front
	cold front
	occluded front
	convergence line: here the wind changes direction — often indicates areas of potential thunderstorm development
1005	isobar line 1005 mbar
NW. 15 kn Ost. 35 kn NO. 20 k	direction and speed of wind in knots: 1 barb equals 10 knots, ½ barb approx. 5 knots
	degree of cloud cover
℞	thunderstorm
	precipitation
	report from a weather station: cloud cover ¾, wind direction NW, wind speed 40 knots

The low

Fronts are a characteristic feature of low-pressure areas in European latitudes. Low-pressure areas move in an easterly direction at a speed of 5 to 45 mph. They absorb the surrounding air, as well as warm air from southern latitudes. According to the laws of physics, the warm air cannot mix with the cold air, so that a warm-air wedge will form, the tip of which reaches into the centre of the low.

When warm and cold air meet on the front and rear edges of this wedge, turbulent zones result, i.e. the warm front and the cold front. The warm air is thus cooled, and can no longer retain its humidity. This results in condensation, i.e. small water droplets appear in the form of clouds. These accumulate into larger drops and then fall as rain.

As a low passes with its fronts, the weather develops as follows: Fine fluffy clouds (cirrostratus) change into milky layer clouds (altostratus), becoming increasingly

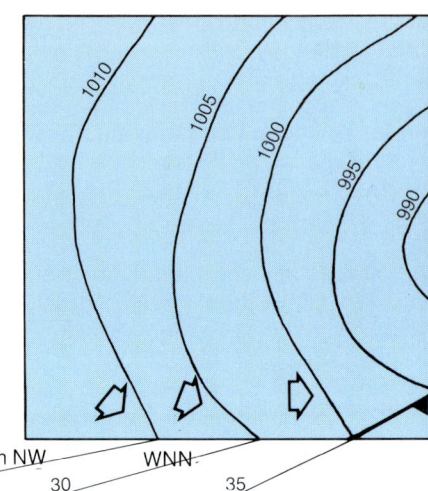

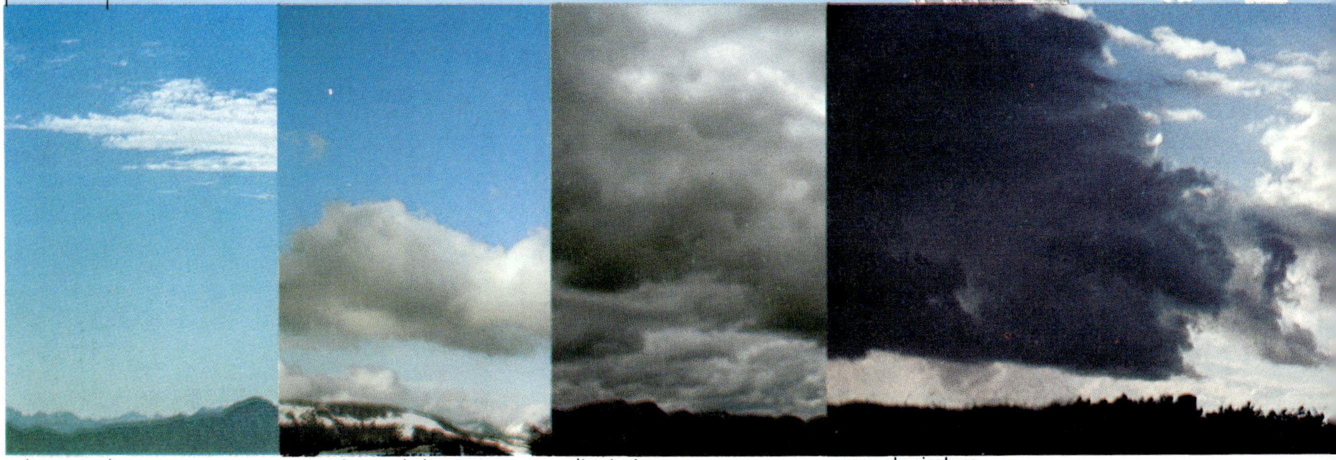

1010 1005 1000 995 990

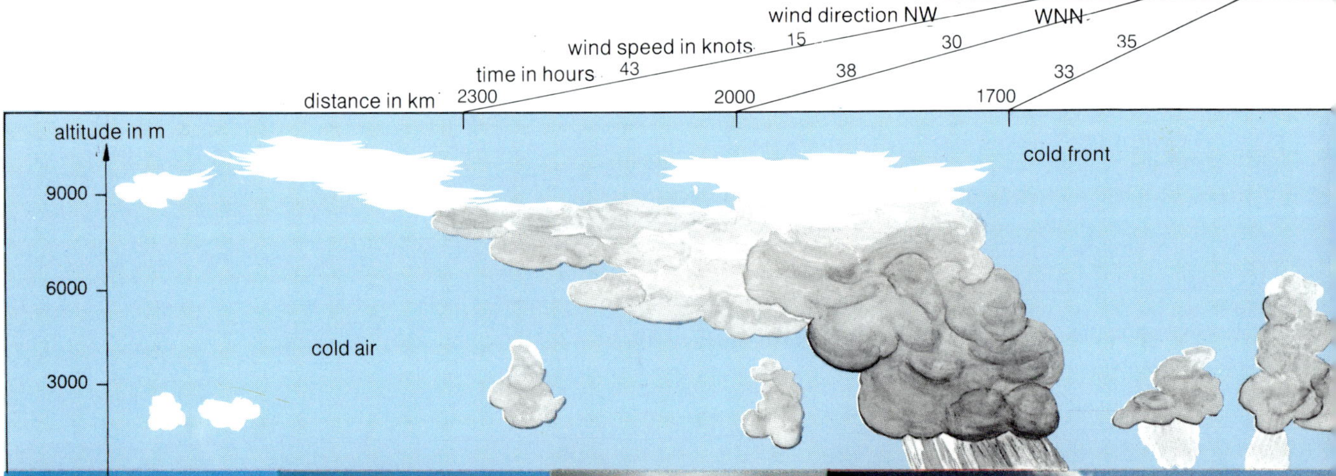

wind direction	NW		WNN	
wind speed in knots	15	30		35
time in hours	43	38		33
distance in km	2300	2000		1700

altitude in m

cold front

9000

6000

cold air

3000

cirrocumulus   cumulus and altostratus   altostratus   cumulonimbus

94

lower and indicating the approach of a warm front. Whereas a south-easterly or south wind blew before the low approached, it now changes its direction to south-west. Finally the warm front arrives in the form of an enormous cloud (the nimbostratus). Even before that, it may start raining steadily, lasting a day or more in most cases. This is followed by the warm sector, in which the rain subsides, the cloud cover breaks up and the atmospheric pressure remains constant.

After one or two days the cold front follows, causing the atmospheric pressure to rise rapidly by a few mbar. Towering heap clouds and westerly squalls of Force 6 to 8 dominate the weather situation. Rain falls in heavy showers and frontal thunderstorms may occur. After a few hours, the cold front has already passed through, so that the cloud cover breaks up again. Temperature and atmospheric pressure rise slowly,

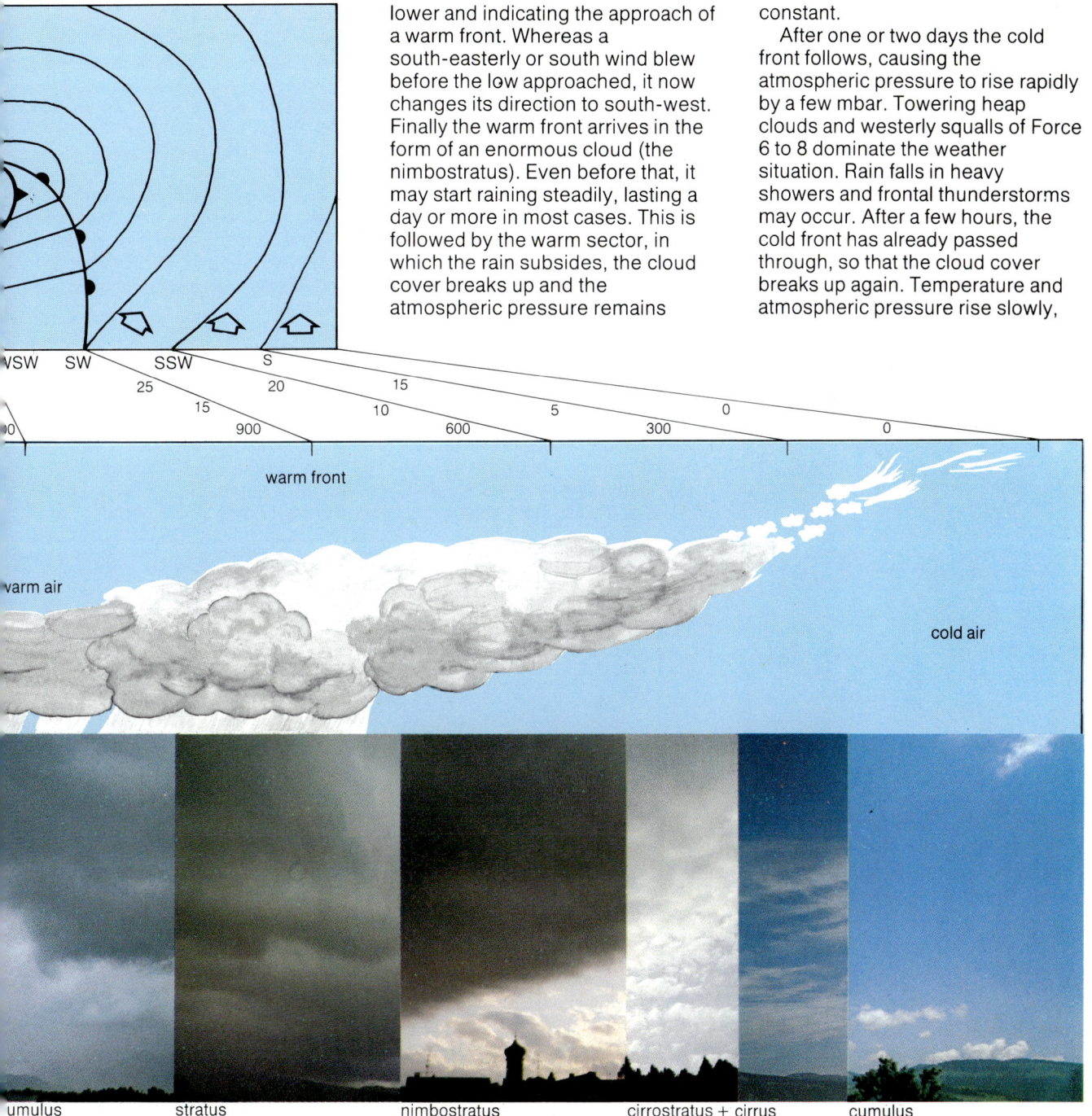

WSW SW   SSW   S
        25   20   15
    15   10   5   0
900   600   300   0

warm front

warm air

cold air

umulus   stratus   nimbostratus   cirrostratus + cirrus   cumulus
                                                        cirrocumulus

95

the wind veers round to the north and dies down. The younger the low is, the more pronounced are the features described. If, however, a low has been travelling for a longer time, the faster-moving cold front will catch up with the warm front and push it upwards, thus creating an occluded front. The weather conditions here resemble those at the cold front. Such occluded lows move only very slowly (5 kn) or stand still. They gradually start to fill so that the pressure gradient evens out and the wind dies down.

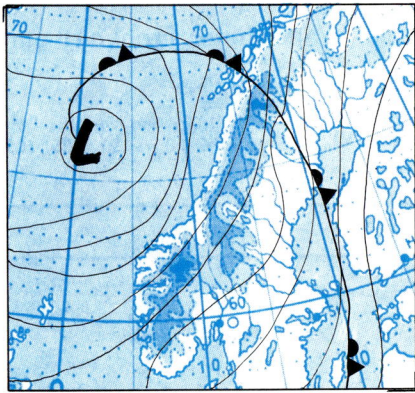

Occluded low over Scandinavia

The high

High-pressure areas produce comparatively calm and stable weather conditions. Rain may fall to the front of a high but as it moves only very slowly, it gives rise to fine stable weather. Thanks to the low pressure gradient winds will be only very weak.

Moreover, high-pressure areas have a controlling effect on the approaching lows. These are deflected around the high.

On or near the land, high-pressure areas can produce local weather conditions. Thermals and convectional thunderstorms arise only in high-pressure areas when the sky is mostly cloudless during the day.

Thermal currents

Thermal currents are produced when air is heated by the sun, becomes lighter and begins to rise. Land heats up faster than water, creating a regular circulation of air on the coast.

Over the land, the air rises, and cooler sea air flows into the gap. On the surface we merely feel the winds near the ground. As it takes a few hours before the land has heated up, this shore breeze does not start blowing until the late morning. It reaches a maximum of Force 3 to 4 in the early afternoon and then dies down again.

During the night, the land cools down faster than the water, which results in the reverse circulation, this time a weaker one. Sometimes, the light offshore wind which now starts to blow can already be felt in the evening.

Because of the irregularly shaped surface of the earth, and because of the pockets of warm air which are continuously re-forming, thermal winds are gusty and often change direction.

Very often thermal winds occur in mountainous regions or in the surrounding areas. During the day the air warms up and rises up the mountainside from the surrounding lowland, so that circulation develops here as well. The valleys act as funnels, sometimes producing winds of Force 6 to 7. Windsurfers

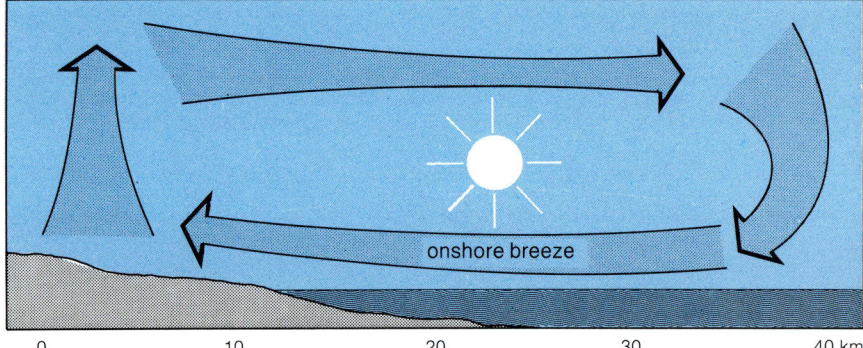

onshore breeze

| 0 | 10 | 20 | 30 | 40 km |

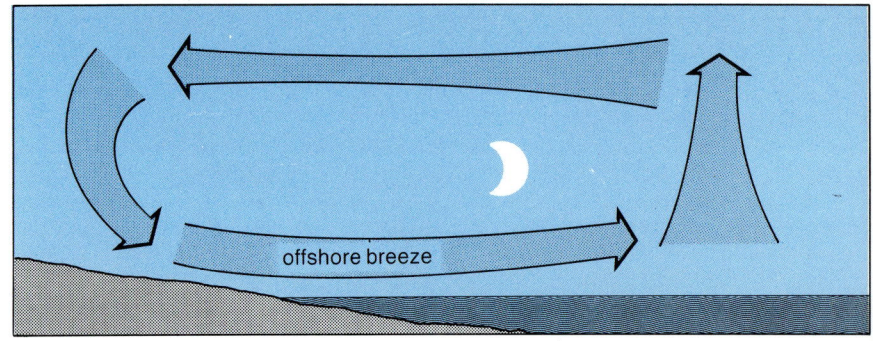

offshore breeze

often meet this phenomenon on Lake Garda in Northern Italy. If the prevailing winds coincide with these local thermal winds, this will increase the wind speed even more. Under the influence of thermal currents, small cumulus clouds or fine-weather clouds will form.

Inversion

Inversion layers act as a kind of brake on the thermal circulations. These are layers of air at a certain altitude which are warmer than the rising thermal. They act like a lid by preventing them from rising any further. Any clouds which form have a well-defined upper boundary. Thermal circulation is not possible and no surface wind will blow. Some radio stations broadcast a daily bulletin of weather reports for gliders, which give precise indications of the altitude and extent of inversion layers.

Thunderstorms

Thunderstorms can be forecast accurately on the basis of measurements. What is more, attentive and observant windsurfers can recognise thunderstorms even before they appear. A dark mushroom-shaped cloud (cumulonimbus) indicates a thunderstorm.

Thunderstorms are triggered off by the vigorous heating of air which has a high level of humidity. The general weather pattern only shows minor pressure differences and the air is relatively cool at higher altitudes. Air which has been heated during the day rises up to meet very cold layers, and suddenly shoots up to altitudes of over six miles. Wind direction and speed are impossible to calculate once a thunderstorm is brewing. The updraught within the cloud tower is Force 5+. Air flows in from all sides, and it is not unusual for it to gust up to Force 8. The energy imbalance within the cloud layers produces electrical charges, which discharge as flashes of lightning. The water droplets which have condensed in the cloud are precipitated as hail or rain. Sometimes the thunderstorm cloud is hidden by haze. Then the only visible sign is the gathering gloom all around. You can tell how far away the thunderstorm is from the time which elapses between the lightning and the thunder. Whereas the sound of the thunder takes about 5 seconds to travel 1 mile, the lightning can be seen immediately.

Therefore, the thunderstorm is 350, 700 or 1050 yards away with a time difference of 1, 2 or 3 seconds respectively. If in spite of all precautions you are caught by a thunderstorm on the open water, crouch down on your board, so that only a small area is exposed to the lightning. Thunderstorms in our latitudes are rarely larger than 6 miles in diameter and in most cases move from SW to NE at between 6 and 12 mph, which means that the storm is usually over in half an hour.

Weather information

In addition to the special weather forecasts for shipping which are provided by the national radio network, it is possible to obtain local weather information over the telephone, or from one of the regional or Public Service Offices of the Meteorological Office.

All the shipping forecasts end with a list of weather reports from coastal stations around the U.K. These are useful for the local weather as are the Inshore Waters Forecasts on BBC Radio 3.

All local radio stations near the coast broadcast information on the nearby coastal waters and you find it best to tune in to the local station nearest your point of operation at about the half-hour past 6, 7 and 8 o'clock and again between 0750 and 0815.

If you are anywhere near a Harbour Master's office you will find an up-to-date forecast is posted up.

Although in the United Kingdom we do not rely on visual signals to tell you about the weather you will sometimes see storm cones hoisted. When you take your board into Europe you will see different warning systems which also indicate the wind direction. If the wind swings round from SE to SW in a low, i.e. it turns clockwise, it is said to *veer*. At other times the wind may turn anti-clockwise, when it is said to *back*.

On lakes, you will find a wide variety of warning systems. Red, orange and white flashing lights on banks are widespread.

It is the duty of every water sportsman to inform himself about the local warning systems. The experienced windsurfer will in any case ask local people or windsurfing schools for details.

wind direction at 4 p.m.

changing wind direction: clock-wise

L (low)

wind direction at 9 a.m.

				The Beaufort Scale		
Bft	kn	mph	m/sec	pressure of wind in kp/m2	name	description
0	–	–	–	–	Calm	Smoke rises vertically; water as smooth as a mirror
1	1–3	1–3	0,3–1,5	0,5–0,3	Light air	Smoke is deflected, ripples
2	4–6	4–7	1,6–3,3	0,3–1	Light breeze	Leaves rustle; small wavelets; smooth crests
3	7–10	8–12	3,4–5,4	1–2	Gentle breeze	Flags move; short waves; occasional white caps
4	11–16	13–18	5,5–8,0	2–5	Moderate breeze	Small branches are moved; white caps fairly general
5	17–12	19–24	8,1–10,7	5–10	Fresh breeze	Wind extends flags; long waves with white caps
6	22–27	25–31	10,8–13,8	10–15	Strong breeze	Large branches in motion; large waves with white crests and spray
7	28–33	32–38	13,9–17,1	15–20	Near gale	Trees in motion; sea heaps up; streaks of foam along the direction of the wind
8	34–40	39–46	17,4–20,7	20–29	Gale	Twigs break off; spray blown from crests of waves
9	41–47	47–54	20,8–24,4	29–44	Severe gale	Slight structural damage; waves topple and roll; spray everywhere
10	48–55	55–63	24,5–28,3	44–59	Storm	Trees uprooted; towering waves; sea white with foam; danger of suffocation in the spray
11	56–65	64--75	28,4–33,5	59–78	Violent storm	Widespread damage; spray hides waves; visibility nil
12	65+	75+	33,5+	78+	Hurricane	Total devastation; air filled with foam and spray

Appendix

Summaries

The following summaries of the chapters on Windsurfing Theory are intended to help you to revise the material and to prepare for the exam.

Boards and equipment

The types of boards used for windsurfing are allround boards, roundboards, funboards, and allround funboards. Funboards are special boards, which are hardly to be recommended for the beginner. Boards differ in length, volume, weight, and the shape of the hull and also in the type of fin and daggerboard which is used. Extreme funboards are called sinkers. Boards which are steered by two sailors are called tandems.

Surfboards are made of thermosetting plastics and thermoplastics. They are filled with different kinds of polyurethane or polystyrene foam.

Surfboards are either made in moulds into which the individual layers are laid, or else they are custom made and are cut and finished from raw foam. One particularly labour-intensive method is the sandwich construction, which is guaranteed to increase the rigidity of the board and save weight.

The parts of the sailing board

are, in addition to the board itself, the fin, the daggerboard, and the rig, which consists of the mast foot, mast, wishbone and sail, plus the ropes and lines with which the sail is tightened, and the uphaul rope.

Daggerboards are made from materials like glassfibre or polypropylene. They come in a variety of shapes. Modern boards have retracting daggerboards which can be swivelled away when they touch bottom or completely retracted when reaching. Others have straight daggerboards. The decisive factor in creating ideal sailing characteristics for a daggerboard is not the size. What is important is the buoyancy it can create. This presupposes a profile which is suited to the speed. Daggerboard and fin prevent the board from moving sideways when beating or reaching. Funboards are often without daggerboards, replacing them with large fins which then assume the function of the daggerboard. There are many forms of fin, such as the big nose, the speed fin, the trapezoid, Kanger's cock and swept back fins. These last two are experimental fins to prevent spin out. They defy all hydrodynamic principles and should therefore, be avoided, as they function like brakes under the board.

Mast foot. In general, for your own safety, each board must be equipped with a safety device which, like ski bindings, releases the mast foot in the event of a potentially dangerous fall. A rubber or universal joint provides a flexible connection between mast foot and mast. The rubber should be as hard as possible.

The mast. Masts are made from materials like Duralumin and various glass-fibre-reinforced plastics. They vary in thickness and stiffness. Masts must match sails in length, thickness and stiffness. A sail will work best when it matches the mast for rigidity.

Beginners are advised to use smaller rigs, which are less demanding in terms of power and technical ability.

The wishbone varies in thickness, rigidity and weight. Its length must match the dimensions of the sail. The distance between clew and aft boom end fitting should be as small as possible when the sail is tightened. Strongwind sailors should make sure that they have rigid wishbone tubes and rigid boom end fittings.

The sail. The edges of the sail are called the luff, leech and foot; the corners are called the head, tack and clew. A sail must have windows, which need to be as large as possible, so that you can see clearly to leeward. The materials used are Dacron and Mylar. Mylar cloth combines almost all the advantages which a sailor could wish to have, such as high speed, low water absorption and no warping. However, Dacron will continue to be the main material for a long time to come, as Mylar is expensive and prone to tearing.

Rig safety line. Every board must have a rig safety line, which keeps board and rig connected if the mast comes away from the board. The rig safety line should form a connection between the nose of the board and the mast foot, so that the board will not tip over and will run with the direction of the current.

The most important accessories are a mast extension and a good uphaul rope. The Hawaiian uphauls, though generally available, are not suitable, as they use up too much strength.

Funboards require foot straps for precise foot steering.

Clothing. Surfing suits are made from Rubatex, neoprene and polyurethane. They are lined with cloth. If you want a tear-proof suit, make sure that it is double bonded.

On the other hand, a single bonded suit keeps you warmer because you sweat less. A decisive factor is the fit of your suit. There should be no chance for water to collect in cavities around the waist. Furthermore, the sleeves must be designed so that the blood can circulate freely.

In winter, dry suits are recommended. Although they do not provide heat themselves (apart from a few exceptions), they may be worn with warm underwear.

Shoes are an indispensable item of equipment for the windsurfer. They prevent your feet from being cut or bruised on the board.

Sailing theory
Directions in relation to the board.
Port tack and starboard tack refer to the relative wind direction. A board which is moving on port tack has its sail to starboard (and vice versa for starboard tack), as the sail is always to leeward. The bow and stern are the front and back end of the board.

Objects in front of a board are ahead, those behind the board are astern. The mid-ship line and anything along it are abeam.

Windward is the side of an object which is pointing towards the wind, leeward is the opposite side.

Steering can mean either heading up or bearing away. Heading up means altering course towards the wind. For this purpose the sail is sheeted in. When you bear away, the board will turn towards a running course. For this the sail is opened out at quite an angle to the board. The direction in which you are steering is called the course. A course may be determined by

reference to a number of different things (such as wind direction). In windsurfing this is related to the wind. Accordingly, some courses are given the following names: beating (which is as close as possible to the wind), beam reach (which is at right angles to the wind), broad reach (meaning at an angle to the wind), and running (which means going in exactly the same direction as the wind). Courses may refer to port tack or starboard tack, i.e. the wind may hit the sail from starboard or port (the sail curves to leeward).

Wind propulsion. Two different principles apply when you are sailboarding: resistance sailing, in which the sail catches the wind and is thus propelled forward; and lift sailing, in which the air has to cover different distances on the inside and outside of the sail, causing a pressure gradient on the sail, which in turn results in a suction effect towards the front of the leeward side. The resulting forces may be assumed to combine in one point, the Centre of Effort. At this point, the forces act almost at right angles to the chord of the sail.

The total force is divided into two components: the driving force and the leeway force. The unwanted leeway force is counteracted by the daggerboard or fin and the part of the board which is underwater. They reduce the sideways displacement of the movement (leeway) on courses which are at an angle to the wind. The leeway force cannot be excluded altogether: the less effective the area of lateral resistance (i.e. the smaller the area presented or the slower the board is moving), the stronger the leeway force.

The sailing wind. When you are travelling on a surfboard, the wind you feel is not the same as the wind which you feel when standing still, the true wind. The wind caused by the movement of the board, makes the apparent wind hit you at more of an angle and with a different speed from that of the true wind. The sail is adjusted to the apparent wind. As the direction of the apparent wind is determined by both the speed of the board and the speed of the true wind, its direction changes whenever one of these two components changes direction. When a gust hits your sail, it will back towards the true wind. When the board accelerates, it will veer towards the bow. When the board slows down, it will return.

Steering. Steering is effected by taking advantage of the difference between the total force and the resistance force. Effective steering with the rig is carried out along the line of the sail: to the front and to windward for bearing away, and to leeward and astern for heading up. Other steering movements can produce unexpected effects, such as inertia on the part of the board or a catapult fall.

The weather and lee helm of a board refer to the board's tendency to head up or bear away while the rig is in its normal position. Funboards without a daggerboard have stronger weather helm when the mastfoot is placed further to the front; boards with a daggerboard would have more lee helm.

Displacing and planing. Some types of surfboards may be called displacers, but they are in fact planers similar to the jollies in sailing. They have the characteristics which justify this classification, as they are too light for displacers. If a boat could only travel as a displacer, it could never leave its wave system, the form of which is determined by the board's length at the water-line. A board 14 feet long could only go at 6 mph. Shorter boards would be even slower.

Seamanship

Ropes. Only synthetic fibres are used for the ropes on surfboards. They do not decay and their ends can be heat-sealed as a protection against fraying. The knots produced by these ropes must have the following characteristics: quick tying, stability and quick and easy untying. These requirements are met by the figure-of-eight knot, the reef knot, the sheet bend, the round turn and two half hitches, the rolling hitch and the bow-line.

Maintenance of the daggerboard. You can keep your board for many years if you follow a few basic rules. The board must be protected against blows. Holes must be mended immediately (if need be with adhesive tape), as water penetrating into the foam would cause irreparable damage. Hair-line cracks in the gelcoat must be filled up. Many types of boards will not stand exposure to ultraviolet rays. For this reason, the boards should be kept in the shade. The daggerboards and fins, as well as the mast and the wishbone, need no maintenance. For your own safety you should check them for cracks. In the daggerboard and fin these occur in the area which protrudes underwater. On a mast, the likely spots are at the bottom end and at the wishbone attachment. The wishbone should be checked at the boom end fittings, the area underneath the cleats, the outhaul line and the area between the ends of the harness line.

The sail is the most fragile part of the surfboard. It should be folded properly at all times, and never left flapping in the wind to dry. If it has to dry in the wind, leave it stretched. Small cracks must be mended immediately. A defective mastfoot must be replaced straight away.

Surfing suits. If you want to make sure your suit lasts a long time, it must be protected against direct sunlight, rinsed regularly and rubbed with talc in the winter. The zip-fasteners should be greased.

Rules

Whilst there are very few rules and regulations as to what you can do and where you may go, please remember that you cannot go sailing on private water without getting permission.

On inland waters such as rivers and canals there may be local byelaws which you must know about and observe. Sailing on reservoirs is usually – if allowed at all – under the control of a Royal Yachting Association club and you should, at all times, speak with the Secretary before assuming that you will be welcome. Likewise, many clubs rent inland waters and, since they are the tenants, will not be pleased to see you unless you have asked permission and paid for a day permit.

Wherever you sail, you will usually find that the International Collision

Regulations – commonly called The Rules of the Road – will apply. Remember that traffic will keep to the right (we are one of the very few countries where road traffic keeps to the left and water traffic ALWAYS keeps to the right).

Except where large craft cannot deviate from the main channel for fear of going aground, power gives way to sail. But on your small board it is always easier for you to get out of the way. Do so by changing course firmly, boldly, and in ample time. As between sailing craft there are three primary rules as to who has to get out of the way of the other.

"When each has the wind on a different side, the vessel which has the wind on the PORT side shall keep out of the way of the other." So a sailing vessel which is on the starboard tack has priority over one on the port tack.

"When both sailing vessels have the wind on the same side, the vessel which is to windward shall keep out of the way of the vessel which is to leeward." So the one which the wind will reach first is the one which must take avoiding action. Yet another rule (which applies both to power and sail) is that an OVERTAKING vessel shall keep clear. Finally, remember that if you cannot see with certainty what the other vessel is doing, or you fear a collision, it is just as much your duty to do something about it. If in doubt, keep clear.

Carrying a board on a car roof.

Remember that a good strong rack, properly secured, is the first requirement.

The board should be tightly strapped with proper straps bow downward and facing forward. The boom can be carried, well padded, on top or underneath the board.

The mast, without sail can be strapped alongside.

If front and rear projections are more than 3′ 6″ they should be clearly marked with a bright red or orange plastic bag or something similar and durable.

And don't forget about insurance for both marine and traffic risks.

Racing

Events consisting of several races are held to establish a winner. The places in the races give scores, which are totalled up at the end. The competitor who has scored the lowest number of points is the winner.

The courses used are triangular and consist of several tacks, reaches and runs.

The start for a race is a flying start. Premature starters must get back behind the starting line, and have no right of way until they have crossed the starting line properly.

The rules for giving way are identical with the statutory regulations. They differ only in the overtaking rules (craft can be overtaken on either side; the craft which is being overtaken may force the opponent who overtakes to windward to sail to windward until the overtaking craft reaches the abeam position), and when boards moving in the same direction overlap when rounding a mark.

If you have broken a rule, you can absolve yourself by executing a 720-degree turn with your board.

Other water sportsmen should not insist on their right of way, and should indicate this fact clearly and promptly, although they need not give way.

Certificates of competence

The Royal Yachting Association offers certificates of proficiency for all kinds of water sports, which we recommend, mostly for reasons of insurance. For boardsailing, there are various certificates. For a list of RYA recognised teaching establishments, apply to the Royal Yachting Association, Victoria Way, Woking, Surrey.

Windsurfing and the environment

Due to the mobility of his board, a windsurfer can go surfing in areas where fauna and flora are otherwise undisturbed. Windsurfing has become increasingly popular, and windsurfers as a whole will become a threat to the environment unless they observe a few rules, such as those which have been worked out by the Nature Conservancy Council.

Do not go near reeds and spawning areas. Do not dump waste in the water or on the beach. Only enter and leave the water at the places marked.

Glossary of Sailing Terms

abeam
at right angles to the centreline of the board

aft
at the back end of the board

apparent wind
the wind resulting from a combination of the true wind and the wind due to the movement of the vessel

astern
behind

backing
pushing the sail forwards into the wind so that the wind blows onto the forward side of the sail, e.g. for an emergency stop

bearing away
moving the board away from the wind, i.e. sailing more downwind

beating
sailing to windward

belaying
fastening a rope around a cleat, pin or bitt

block
nautical word for a pulley wheel

bond
coat of a special texture or plastic which is applied on neoprene or similar materials

boom end fitting
fitting where the ends of the wishbone meet

bow
front end of craft (see nose)

buoyancy
the board's ability to float due to the displacement of water (the buoyancy equals the weight of the water which is displaced by a body)

calm
no wind

camber
the curve in the sail, the belly of the sail

cavitation
see spin out

Centre of Buoyancy
the point upon which the upward forces seem to act

Centre of Effort (CE)
the point upon which the wind seems to act

Centre of Lateral Resistance (CLR)
the point upon which the underwater forces seem to act

chord
imaginary line between the two boom end fittings

clew
outer corner of the sail

collision course
course which would lead to a collision

course
the direction a surfboard takes; in the case of sailboarding, mostly refers to the position in relation to the wind, e.g. reaching

custom made
a special type of production: the board is made individually, according to the wishes of the customer

daggerboard
board underneath the surfboard which is specially shaped to reduce the leeway force

displacement barrier
the highest speed which a boat can reach when it is displacement sailing

ebb
see low water

edge of sail
luff, leech, foot

elevation
the hull profile of a boat or a board

emergency gybe
a near emergency stop followed by veering off and shifting the sails

evaporation due to cold
coldness, resulting from the loss of body heat when water on the skin evaporates

eyelet (cringle)
ring made of solid material (brass or plastic), which prevents the trim holes in the sail from tearing or fraying

fairway
navigable channel for ships, which can often only be recognised on a chart

flapping
loose swaying of the sail

flood
see high water

foot
the bottom edge of the sail

freestyle
acrobatics on the surfboard

gust
sudden rush of wind

gybing
changing the side of the sail before the wind

head
top corner of the sail

head to wind
the angle to the wind where the sail cannot produce any forward drive (approx. 45 degrees on port or starboard bow)

heading up
moving the board to windward, i.e. sailing up towards the wind

high water
the period when the tide is in (opposite: low water)

laminate
the outer skin of the board, made from fibre mats which have been soaked in synthetic resin

land breeze
thermal wind blowing from land to sea at night

lateral view
a side view of the underwater area of board, daggerboard and skeg

leech
the rear edge of the sail

lee helm
the tendency of board to bear away/off (the ship carries lee helm)

leeward
the side of an object away from the wind or the space nearby

leeway
lateral off-course movement of a craft under way, which is caused by winds or currents

low water
the period when the tide is out (opposite: high water)

luff
the front edge of the sail

luffing
bringing the board's bow nearer to the wind

mast foot well
the point where the mast is attached to the board

nose (see bow)
front end of a craft

obligation to hold course
the obligation for the sailor who has right of way to continue his course straight ahead

offshore wind
the wind blows off the land towards the sea. Be careful! You will be blown away from the shore, unable to manoeuvre

onshore wind
the wind is blowing from the water onto the land

overlap
two boats overlap when the after boat has crossed an imaginary line drawn at a right angle to the stern of the leading boat

part
a portion of a line

perch
a pole marking the waterway. The trunk of a young tree, the top of which marks starboard or port

plane of sail
area which projects vertically above and below the chord

planing
skimming through the water with buoyancy and minimum displacement, thus breaking the displacement barrier

port
the left side of a craft, left

port tack
when making headway the wind is on the port side of the craft

railriding
steering the board by shifting one's weight

reaching
course which is at 90° to the wind

real wind
see true wind

reeving
passing a rope through an opening, e.g. in a pulley (see block)

rig
mast, sail, wishbone and other equipment necessary for propulsion

rig safety line
short line with which the mast is leashed to the board

rig steering
steering by raking the rig

rigging up
assembling the rig, i.e. sail, mast, wishbone and accessories, so that it is ready to sail

rocker
the curve in the fore and aft part of a board

roundboard
a large-volume surfboard, which shows ideal displacement characteristics at low speeds

scoop
see rocker

sea breeze
thermal wind blowing from sea to land by day

sheeting in
hauling the sail in, i.e. more parallel to the board

shoal
shallow place in the sea

shock cord
an elasticated cord which connects the uphaul rope to the mast foot

spin out
turbulence from the fin at high speeds, causing the board to turn sideways

starboard
right side of a craft; on the right side

starboard tack
when making headway the wind is on the starboard side of the craft

submarining
involuntary diving of the bow into the water

tack
lower forward corner of the sail

tack
when beating up, the distance between two turning points

tacking
altering course when sailing close-hauled by shifting the sail from starboard to port with the bow to windward (or vice versa)

tail
the back end of the board

tide
period of time lasting 12 hours 25 minutes, during which one flood tide and one ebb tide take place

towing line, towing eye
accessories needed for rescue.

trimming
trying to find the ideal position for the board and the sail

true wind
the wind actually blowing

weather helm
the tendency of a board to head up (the ship carries weather helm)

wind shadow
the area which is sheltered from the wind by an obstacle, and in which the wind may blow gently in different directions. Be careful! You may misjudge the wind when it blows offshore

windward
the side of, and the area in front of, an object towards which the wind is blowing

windward barrier effect
an area in front of an obstacle in which the wind pressure drops

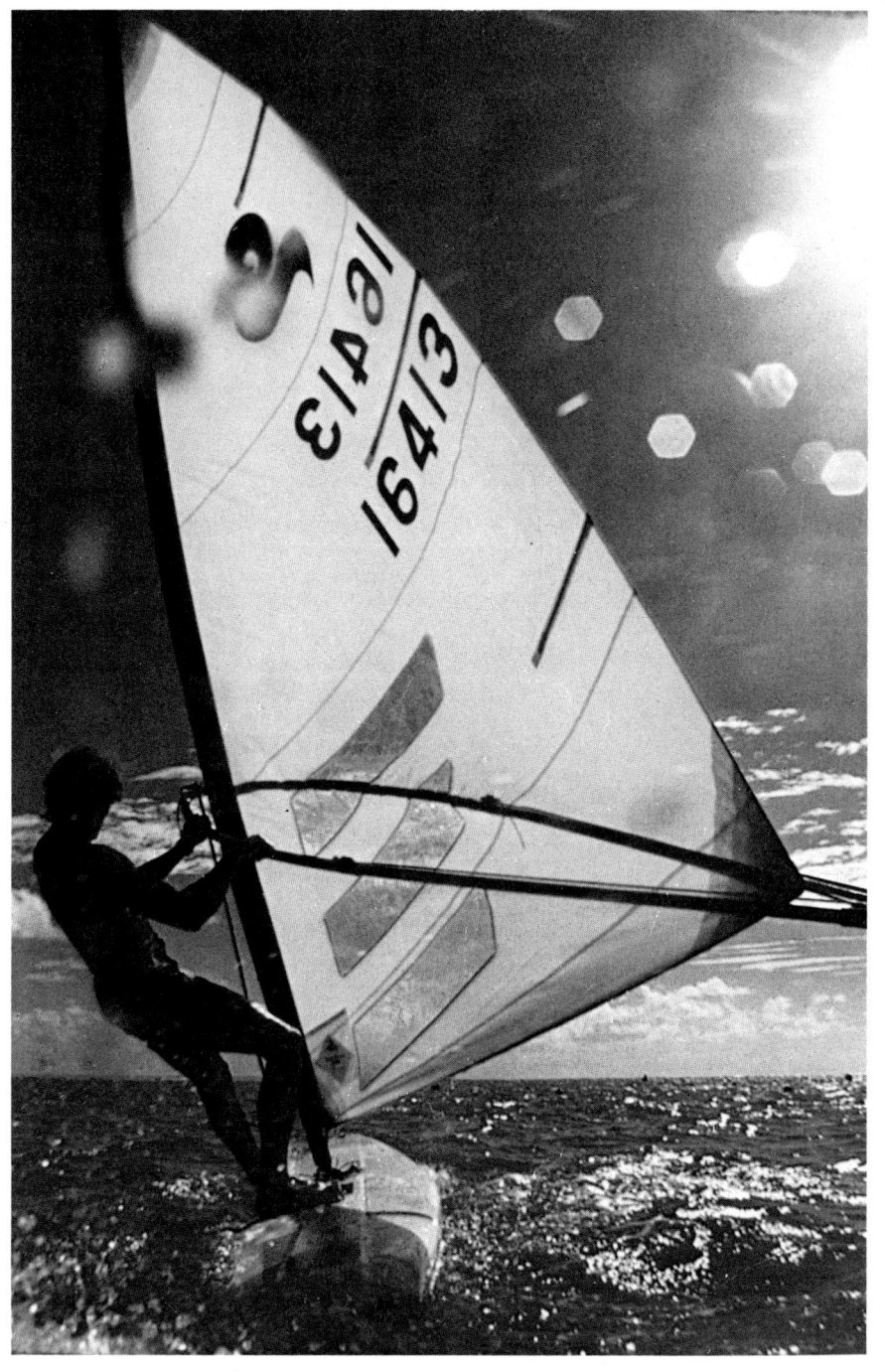

Test Questions

Windsurfing in Practice

How do you get your rig round from windward to leeward in order to pull up the sail:
a) if you want to carry on in the same direction?

● Pull the rig over the bow or stern.

b) if you want to change direction?

● Lift the rig slightly and let the wind blow you round.

What movements do you need to make to sheet in and luff?

● Turn the upper part of your body.

Why is the emergency stop the most useful way of stopping?

● Because the board comes to a halt in the shortest possible distance, and it remains manoeuvrable.

On what courses is the emergency stop not possible?

● When running or on a broad reach.

What movements of the rig make the board
a) head up?

● Tilting the rig to leeward along the line of the sail.

b) bear off?

● Tilting the rig to windward along the line of the sail.

Which edge of the board must you put your weight on in order to bear off more sharply in the case of a board fitted with a daggerboard?

● The windward edge.

What are the advantages of a fast turn over a normal turn?

● You make a lot of headway against the wind.
● You move to the opposite side of the sail as quickly and safely as possible.

What are the advantages of a fast gybe over a normal gybe?

● You do not lose much headway against the wind.
● You move to the opposite side of the sail as quickly and safely as possible.

Under what circumstances should you not use the beach start for safety reasons?

● When the beach is rocky.
● When the ground drops away sharply.
● When there are a lot of people on the beach.

How would you describe the correct sail position for practical purposes?

● The sail is sheeted in just far enough to stop it flapping.

What is the most important requirement for surfing without using too much energy?

● Keeping the sail in the correct position.

Give three reasons why windsurfers keep getting into difficulties at sea.

● Wrong or damaged equipment.
● Overestimating their abilities.
● Unfamiliarity with the area.

What is the point of a harness?

● It makes it possible for the skilled surfer to carry on sailing for a longer time.
● It provides a safety reserve for emergencies.

What should you expect of a good harness line?

● It should be possible to hook on and unhook without taking your hands off the wishbone.
● It should have one or more quick-release buckles.

Describe two emergency signals.

● Stretching your arms out sideways and raising and lowering them.
● Releasing a red distress flare or orange smoke signal.

What are the four possible ways of towing?

● Towing with a bar, with a rope, by the daggerboard strap or footstrap, and with the rig trailing.

Why is it easier to tow a board from which the daggerboard has been removed?

● Because the board being towed no longer has any tendency to steer itself.

Boards and Equipment

Name three different types of surfboards.

● Allround boards, roundboards, funboards, allround funboards.

Name two design features of a roundboard.

● Large rocker on the nose, high volume.

Name two design features of a funboard.

● Flat bottom for planing, low volume, strong scoop, no daggerboard.

Name the features of an allround funboard.

● Flat bottom for planing, board length approx. 11 ft. 6 in., retracting or sickle-shaped daggerboard.

What materials are used for making surfboards?

● Duroplastics (epoxy and polyester resins) and thermoplastics (polyethylene, ABS and ASA).

How do you repair polyethylene?

● With hot air welding equipment or a soldering iron. Only a professional should carry out repairs.

Name three types of foam which are used for making surfboards.

● Polyurethane foam, polystyrene foam, phenolic foams.

Name two methods of producing surfboards.

● Hand-layer method, custom made construction, blow-moulding.

Describe the individual steps involved in the custom made board construction.

● Cut and grind the foam block. Then laminate the foam and trim excess foam by hand.

What is the meaning of a) rocker, b) scoop?

● a) The curvature in the aft plane of the board.
 b) The curvature at the nose of the board.

Name a few types of daggerboards.

● Straight daggerboard, storm daggerboard, swivel daggerboard, retracting daggerboard.

Name a few different types of fins.

● Big nose fin, speed fin, trapezoid fin, Kanger's cock fin, pin tail fin.

Name two different mast foot joints.

● Universal joint (UJ), rubber joint.

What is the typical feature of a mast foot?

● It should include a release device which can be adjusted very precisely.

What is the function of the rig safety line?

● It keeps board and rig together if the mast foot comes out of the mast foot well. This prevents the board from drifting away.

Where do you fix the rig safety line?

● Its front end is fixed to the bow. The other end is fastened to the mast foot.

Why is it not advisable to buy soft mast foot joints?

● They tend to tear, i.e. they constitute a safety risk. They also warp under strain and prevent accurate handling of the rig.

Name a few criteria which are important to consider when buying a mast.

● Mast and sail must match. The mast should be easy to handle, i.e. it should be light and thin in diameter.

What materials are masts made of?

● Aluminium, reinforced glass fibre, and epoxy resin.

Name the parts of the wishbone.

● The aluminium tube and boom end fittings.

What should you bear in mind when buying a wishbone?

● The rigidity of the tube, the solid rubber cover, firmly fastened cleats. The wishbone should not be too heavy and its length should match the size of the sail.

What happens when you are sailing in strong winds with a soft wishbone?

● The wishbone will stretch and the Centre of Effort in the sail will change. This means that precise steering is impossible.

Name the edges and corners of the sail.

● The edges are luff, leech and foot; the corners are head, tack and clew.

What is the purpose of the window?

● A sufficiently large window enables the surfer to observe the traffic around him and especially leeward craft and swimmers.

What equipment is used to trim the sail?

● The outhaul line near the clew, the downhaul line near the tack, and the adjustment of the wishbone in the mast sleeve gap.

What materials are surfing sails made of?

● Dacron and Mylar cloth.

What are the advantages of Mylar over Dacron?

● Mylar does not stretch or twist, which makes it possible to determine the profile from the very beginning; no air can penetrate and practically no water can get into it.

Why is it not a good idea to equip a funboard with a sail with a normal low clew?

● The aft end of the wishbone will dip into the sea at high speeds because the mast is so far forward.

Why is it not a good idea to sail an allround board with a sail with a high clew?

● The gap between foot and board becomes too large, which results in the pressure between leeward and windward side of the sail being equalised. This will decrease speed.

With what accessory is it possible to adjust the wishbone above the head when the mast sleeve gap for the wishbone is positioned too low?

● By inserting a mast extension.

Why should a funboard only be equipped with the necessary number of footstraps?

● Footstraps are not required at low speeds. Furthermore, they hinder the surfer when he has to change position.

What materials are surfing suits made of?

● From neoprene, Rubatex, Freetex, and other polyurethane materials.

What is the function of the surfing shoe?

● It protects the foot from injuries when stepping down from the board on the beach and from toe injuries on the board.

Sailing Theory

Where are port and starboard on a surfboard?

● Port is on the left, starboard on the right.

Draw a surfboard which is going a) on starboard tack, b) on port tack.

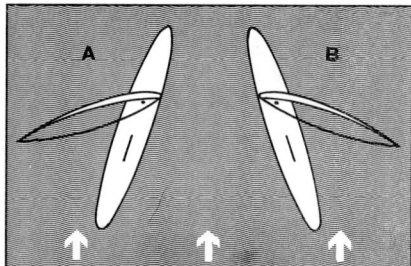

Draw a buoy which is a) abeam, b) right ahead of a surf board.

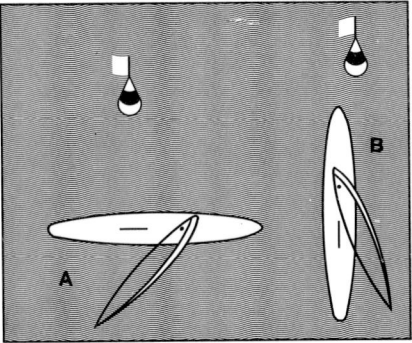

Mark the windward and leeward sides on a surfboard.

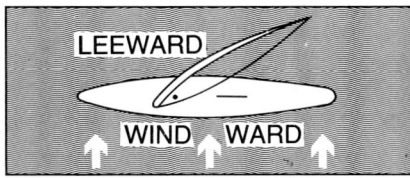

What do "head up" and "bear away" mean in windsurfing?

● Heading up means altering course to windward; bearing away means changing to leeward.

Show the sail position of a surfboard which is beating.

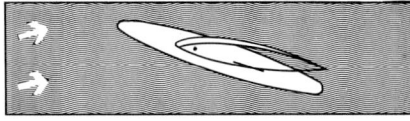

What is the sail's position in relation to the board when running?

● It is at right angles to the board.

Up to approximately what angle in relation to the wind can you make headway on your board?

● Up to approximately 45 degrees.

Why is it possible for a surfboard to go at an angle to the wind?

● This is due to the lateral resistance underwater.

What is leeway and how can you reduce it?

● Leeway is the side displacement of a surfboard in motion. It can be reduced if the lateral plane or the speed is increased.

When should special attention be paid to the leeway?

● On beating courses and when moving at low speed.

Mark the true wind, the wind due to the movement of the board and the apparent wind as they affect a surfboard.

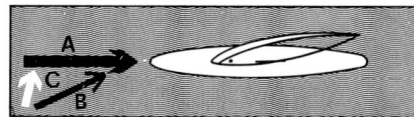

a) wind due to the movement of board
b) apparent wind
c) true wind

When do the directions of the apparent and the true wind coincide?

● On a running course.

What effect does apparent wind have when you are travelling in gusty winds?

● In a gust, the apparent wind backs towards the direction of the true wind (hauls backward); when the board accelerates, it veers towards the front again (hauls forward).

Why is a surfboard accelerated in front of a wave and how does the apparent wind interfere?

● The current created at the front end of the wave accelerates the board. The wind hauls forward.

Mark the directions of the wind and resistance forces acting on a surfboard above and below the waterline.

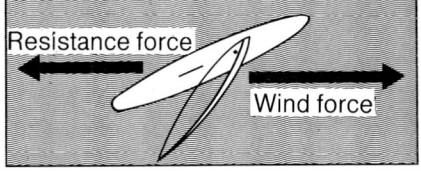

How can you raise a funboard's weather helm?

● The mastfoot has to be shifted towards the bow, the fins must be moved further to the front.

How can you increase the weather helm on a board with a daggerboard?

● The mastfoot is moved towards the stern.

Seamanship

Name the materials from which ropes are made.

● Natural fibres and plastics.

What has to be done to prevent the ropes from fraying?

● A rope end protection must be put on the ends. Synthetic ropes are heat-sealed (welded rope end protection).

What are the characteristics of woven ropes and why are they used almost exclusively in windsurfing?

● Woven ropes are very flexible and hold better in the cleats than twisted material.

Name the advantages of synthetic ropes as compared to natural fibres.

● Synthetic fibres are very resistant to fracture and do not decay.

What are the qualities a seaman's knot must have?

● A seaman's knot must be easy to tie and untie. It must also be very stable.

What is the following knot called? Give an example of where you can use it.

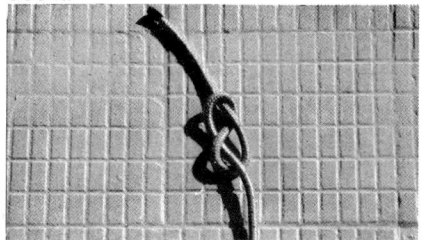

● It is called a figure-of-eight knot. It can be used, for example, as means to secure the rope behind a cleat.

What is the following knot called and where can it be used?

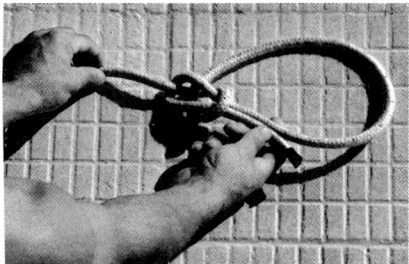

● It is a bowline. It serves as a noose which cannot be tightened. It is used to fix the outhaul line to the clew.

Where do you tie a rolling hitch?

● To attach the inhaul to the mast.

Why do you have to mend any hole in your board immediately?

● Water penetrating the foam in the board cannot be removed and destroys the structure of the cells. When the board gets hot, it also separates the foam from the outer skin.

Why do we recommend that you get off your board as soon as the water reaches knee depth?

● This avoids the danger of your hitting the ground and falling off. Furthermore, it means that you are handling the board, daggerboard and fin with care.

At which points on a windsurfing mast can you expect fracture points?

● At the wishbone attachment and at the lower end.

What are the most common fracture points on a wishbone?

● They are the boom end fittings and the area between the ends of the harness line.

List some measures which serve to prolong the life of your sail.

● Always fold the sail when it is dry. Avoid folds on the window. If possible, dry the sail in a place where there is no wind. Loosen the trimming lines.

Why do you have to repair even minor splits in the sail at once?

● The high pressure applied to the sail would otherwise quickly make them into large holes.

Why should you replace a torn mastfoot rubber as soon as possible?

● A defective rubber is a safety risk.

How can you prolong the life of your surfing suit?

● *It must be rinsed regularly after use. Direct sunlight must be avoided when it is drying, and it should be stored carefully during the winter.*

Rules

Can a boardsailor sail on private water?

● Only after getting permission.

Which side of the river would a pleasure steamer be likely to sail?

● The right hand side.

Why should you obtain information about an inland water with which you are not familiar?

● Many waters are subject to byelaws or other special regulations.

What qualifications is it advisable to have in order to use a sailboard?

● One of the Royal Yachting Association's certificates of proficiency.

List three areas where you would not take your sailboard.

● Marked bathing areas.
● The navigation channels for big ships.
● Where birds or fish may be breeding.

What is the correct name for the Rules of the Road?

● The International Regulations for Preventing Collisions at Sea.

If you think a collision is likely and the other craft does not appear to be taking any action what should you do?

● Change course to avoid the collision and do it firmly, boldly and in ample time to make the intention clear.

If there is a danger of collision would you a) Turn away b) Try to speed up to cross in front of the other vessel c) Go behind him (i.e. pass under his stern)?

● a) or c) is always the answer. (b) is just asking for trouble.

List three rules of the road which apply as between sailing vessels.

● The vessel which is on starboard has priority.
● The vessel which is to windward must keep clear.
● The overtaking vessel must keep clear.

Draw surfboards on port tack and starboard tack which are on a collision course. Who has to give way?

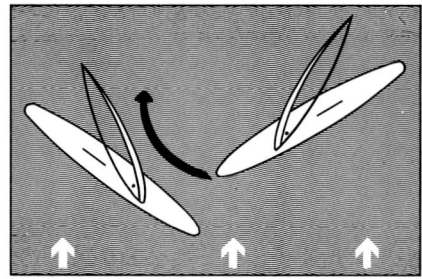

● The boat which is on port tack.

Who has to give way when a motor-operated small vessel and a sailing vessel are on a collision course?

● The motor-operated small vessel has to give way. It passes behind the stern of the sailing vessel, if at all possible.

How can leeward and windward be defined?

● Leeward is the side on which the sail is.

What is the order of priority in this drawing?

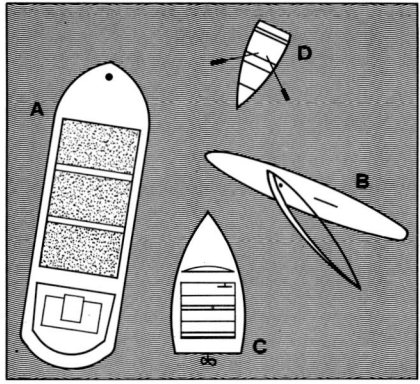

● A–B–D–C
The large barge is obviously in a narrow channel and cannot move aside for fear of grounding.
The sailboard is under sail and has priority over small self-propelled craft.
And power gives way to sail so C has the least priority.

Having established the priority of A–B–C–D in the diagram it is clear that collision is inevitable. What should you have done LONG before the situation developed?

- Although you have priority over the rowing boat and the small launch it is quite clear that you would have been, much earlier, in a position to tack and keep clear of what was obviously going to be a tricky situation. You should not even be in the diagram!

Is a yacht under engine a sailing boat or a power-driven vessel?

- When under power a yacht must act as a power-driven vessel even though its sails may still be hoisted. Whilst it may be difficult for a boardsailor to tell this his duty is to maintain his course. The yacht under power should give way – "Power gives way to sail" – but if it does not then it is no good maintaining your course and speed until a collision occurs. Your duty would be, perhaps at the last minute, to do an emergency stop and certainly to alter course.

If you saw a boardsailor kneeling on his board and raising and lowering his outstretched arms what would you do?

- Since everybody is obliged by law to help somebody in distress if he can, you should go to him and perhaps assist him by towing him in?

If you saw a motor yacht on fire what would you do?

- You obviously cannot render much assistance and the intelligent thing to do would be to sail as fast as you can to the shore and summon assistance, preferably by telling the Coastguard by 'phone or in person.

What other emergency signals do you know other than the signal with the arms and a red distress flare?

- These are listed in the International Collision Regulations but we have mentioned an orange smoke flare.

Where can you obtain information on the regulations which apply to the area?

- From the harbour office, the local sailing and surfing clubs, and the local people.

How do you react when you are confronted with a vessel with restricted draught?

- Its free passage must not be obstructed.

If you came across a fishing vessel which was obviously fishing what would you do?

- Keep a sharp eye out for obstructions on the surface and keep away from him.

If you saw a green buoy rather like the one in the diagram what would you deduce from it?

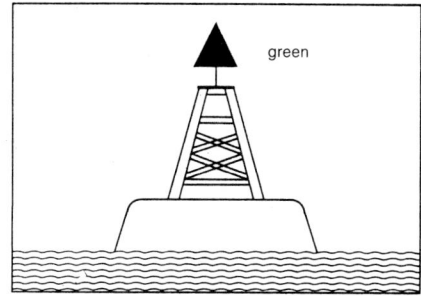

- Green buoys mark the right hand side of a main channel from seaward and the deduction would be that you were about to enter a shipping channel.

What would be your next action in such circumstances?

- The correct action would be to alter course so that you kept out of the shipping channel.

What colour and shape would the buoy on the other side of the channel be?

- Red, and its shape or top mark would be square.

List as many points about carrying a board on a roof-rack as you can remember.

- strong rack – properly secured.
- Tight straps of the right kind.
- Bow of board downward and facing the front, preferably secured to the front bumper.
- Boom well padded.
- Rear projection marked with bright red or orange material especially if more than 3′ 6″.
- Check insurance for marine and traffic purposes.

Racing

What is the International body which makes the racing rules called?

● The International Yacht Racing Union.

What is the National Authority of the sport of racing yachts and boards in the United Kingdom?

● The Royal Yachting Association.

When would you expect the Blue Peter to be hoisted and when would it be lowered when racing was in progress?

● It would be hoisted five minutes before the start of the race.
● It would be lowered at the moment when the race starts.

What is the blue and white (chess-board) flag called and what does it mean?

● It is called Flag "N" of the International Code of Signals and for racing it means "Race abandoned".

When would Flag "S" be used during the management of a race?

● When, for reasons such as bad weather, or no wind, the race officials wish to shorten the course.

What would you hear if you were over the line at the start of a race?

● One gun in addition to the starting gun.

What is a regatta?

● A series of races to establish the regatta winner.

What is the correct behaviour of premature starters, who are recalled by the start vessel?

● They must return to the starting area and must give way to the other boards until they have crossed the starting line properly.

What is the meaning of "abeam"?

● On a line at right angles to the middle of the ship's centreline.

Define the terms "clear ahead", to "overlap", and "clear astern".

● A board is *clear astern*, when it is sailing behind an imaginary line drawn at right angles to the tail of another board. The other board is *clear ahead*. If the aft board has crossed this line, then it is called an *overlap*.

What is the correct behaviour for one competitor towards the other competitors during a manoeuvre?

● He has to keep clear during the manoeuvre.

How can a competitor absolve himself after causing a collision?

● By executing a 720-degree turn.

What is the correct behaviour of a competitor towards other water sportsmen who are not racing?

● He has to observe the "Rules of the Road."

You have got into a regatta area. Which rules of giving way apply? What will be your behaviour?

● The normal rules for giving way are in effect. You should try to leave the area immediately.

What do the sail insignia include?

● The class insignia, the boat/board number, and the nationality sign.

Name a few variations of windsurfing.

● Racing, freestyle, funboard surfing, tandem surfing.

Name at least four areas into which you should not intrude with your surfboard if you want to help the environment.

● Reeds, spawning areas, bird sanctuaries, seal colonies.

What is the minimum distance you should keep away from reeds?

● At least 30 to 50 yards.

What is the correct behaviour when you encounter flocks of birds on water or land?

● Keep a distance of at least 100 yards.

The weather

When and where would you inquire about local conditions before sailing?

● Before taking to the water, at the harbourmaster's office, the local club and/or any local school or clubs connected with windsurfing or sailing.

What sources of information do you know for enquiring about the weather?

● TV and radio stations, telephone services, weather stations, and (sometimes) airforce stations.

What does a cumulonimbus cloud look like (altitude, form, colour)?

● It billows up like an enormous mushroom, penetrating all the cloud layers up to approx. 30,000 ft; its lower part is dark, often with irregular squall clouds; the upper part is white (with ice crystals).

What sort of weather does cumulonimbus indicate?

● The danger of thunderstorms; when it approaches, stormy winds of up to force 8 from variable directions; rain and hail.

How far away is a thunderstorm, when 6 seconds elapse between lightning and thunder?

● 6÷5 = approx. 1⅕ miles

What changes in air pressure do you expect when
a) a high forms?
b) a low is approaching?

● a) slow, continuous increase in pressure
  b) sudden and rapid drop in pressure.

In our latitudes, with westerly winds, each young low contains a wedge of warm air. Give the names and symbols on a weather chart for the front and rear edges of this warm air sector, and describe its position in relation to the centre of the low.

● The warm front forms the front edge; ⌒⌒
the cold front forms the rear edge; ▷◁
the wedge is located to the south of the low, with the tip pointing to the centre.

What is the meaning of these symbols on a weather chart?

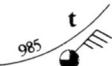

t	= a trough
985	= barometric pressure 985 mbar along the isobar
◗	= 3/4 cloud cover
⟪	= NE wind, force 7

Describe three different fronts which may occur in low pressure areas and draw their respective symbols.

● Warm front: low, dark rain clouds, steady rain, wind veering;

● Cold front: dark wall of clouds with heavy showers, wind strengthens and veers;
● Occluded front: cold front has undercut warm front: it is like a weak cold front.

What are isobars, and what can you conclude from the direction and pressure of the wind?

● Isobars are lines which indicate places of equal pressure; the direction of the wind is at 15 degrees to the isobars. The closer the isobars are together, the higher the pressure gradient and the higher the wind speed.

Describe the effects in western latitudes of an approaching warm front on:
a) the direction and speed of the wind
b) barometric pressure
c) temperature
d) the cloud pattern
e) precipitation

● a) wind strengthens and veers
  b) pressure decreases
  c) temperature remains steady for the time being and immediately afterwards increases slightly
  d) the clouds become lower and lower
  e) light but steady rain

Tides

What do you understand by high and low water?

● high water/tide is the highest water level of a tide,
low water/tide is the lowest water level of a tide.

How long does a tide last from high tide to high tide (i.e. one full flood and one ebb)?

● 12½ hours

At what time does the strongest current occur during a tide?

● At the mid-point between high and low tide.

How far can tidal currents in narrows carry a windsurfer within 15 minutes?

● Up to 1½ miles.

What unexpected effects may the tides have on the currents?

● An increase or a reversal in current due to narrows or the configuration of the coast line.

You see the following line in a tide table:
17 F O 0.24 12.38 7.05 19.36 HW LW
What is the meaning of the letters and figures?

● 17th day of the month; Friday; new moon; high water times: 0024 and 1238; low water times: 0705 and 1936.

You will find the following data for Rantum Bay in the tide table:
HW + 2.33 LW + 2.33.
What do they mean?

● High water and low water times are 2 hours 33 minutes later than the nearest principal port.

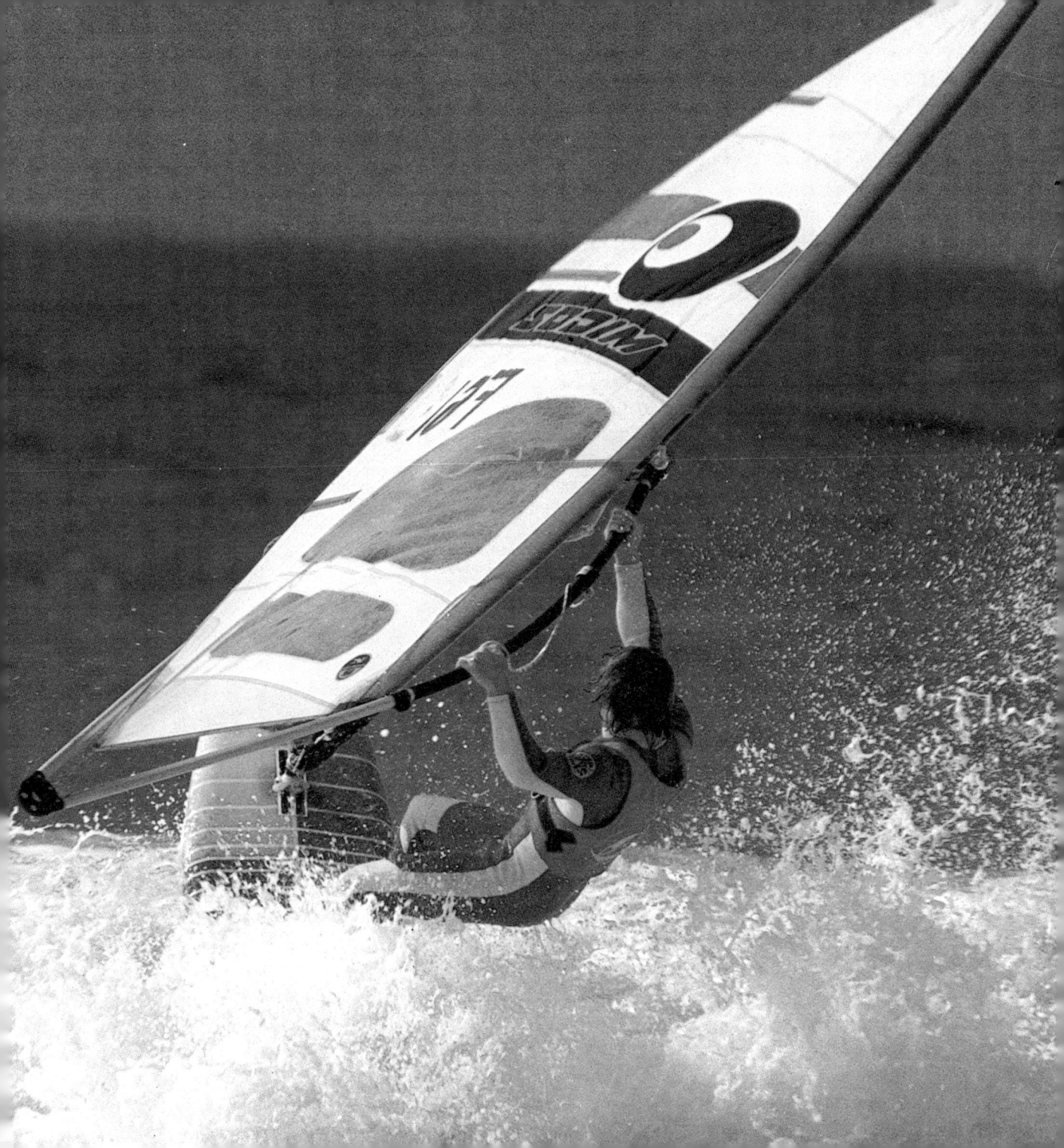

Index